CBT EXPRESS

Also Available

*Clinical Practice of Cognitive Therapy with Children and Adolescents,
Second Edition: The Nuts and Bolts*
Robert D. Friedberg and Jessica M. McClure

*Cognitive Therapy Techniques for Children and Adolescents:
Tools for Enhancing Practice*
Robert D. Friedberg, Jessica M. McClure,
and Jolene Hillwig Garcia

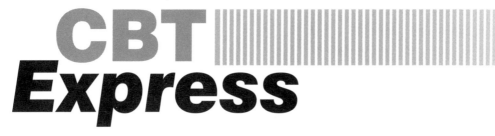

CBT
Express

Effective 15-Minute Techniques
for Treating Children and Adolescents

Jessica M. McClure
Robert D. Friedberg
Micaela A. Thordarson
Marisa Keller

Foreword by Judith S. Beck

THE GUILFORD PRESS
New York   London

Copyright © 2019 The Guilford Press
A Division of Guilford Publications, Inc.
370 Seventh Avenue, Suite 1200, New York, NY 10001
www.guilford.com

Printed in the United States of America

This book is printed on acid-free paper.

Last digit is print number: 9   8   7   6   5   4   3   2   1

The authors have checked with sources believed to be reliable in their efforts to provide
information that is complete and generally in accord with the standards of practice that are
accepted at the time of publication. However, in view of the possibility of human error or
changes in behavioral, mental health, or medical sciences, neither the authors, nor the editor
and publisher, nor any other party who has been involved in the preparation or publication
of this work warrants that the information contained herein is in every respect accurate or
complete, and they are not responsible for any errors or omissions or the results obtained from
the use of such information. Readers are encouraged to confirm the information contained in
this book with other sources.

Library of Congress Cataloging-in-Publication Data is available from the publisher.

ISBN 978-1-4625-4030-3 (paperback)
ISBN 978-1-4625-4031-0 (hardcover)

Illustrations by Rosa Pogessi.

About the Authors

Jessica M. McClure, PsyD, is Clinical Director of the Division of Behavioral Medicine and Clinical Psychology at Cincinnati Children's Hospital Medical Center. Dr. McClure has presented, written articles and book chapters, and provided training in cognitive-behavioral therapy with children and adolescents, including those with anxiety, depression, and behavioral disorders. She is coauthor of *Clinical Practice of Cognitive Therapy with Children and Adolescents, Second Edition: The Nuts and Bolts*, and *Cognitive Therapy Techniques for Children and Adolescents: Tools for Enhancing Practice*.

Robert D. Friedberg, PhD, ABPP, is Full Professor and Head of the Child Emphasis Area at Palo Alto University. Previously, he directed the CBT Clinic for Children and Adolescents and the Psychology Postdoctoral Fellowship Program at Penn State Health Milton S. Hershey Medical Center. Dr. Friedberg served as an Extramural Scholar at the Beck Institute for Cognitive Behavior Therapy and is a Fellow of both the American Psychological Association (Society of Clinical Child and Adolescent Psychology) and the Association for Behavioral and Cognitive Therapies. He is coauthor of *Clinical Practice of Cognitive Therapy with Children and Adolescents, Second Edition: The Nuts and Bolts*, and *Cognitive Therapy Techniques for Children and Adolescents: Tools for Enhancing Practice*.

Micaela A. Thordarson, PhD, is Program Supervisor of the adolescent intensive outpatient program at Children's Hospital of Orange County in Orange, California. Dr. Thordarson supervises trainees in the implementation of cognitive-behavioral interventions across a variety of clinical contexts.

Marisa Keller, PhD, is a clinical psychologist on the cognitive-behavioral therapy and dialectical behavior therapy (DBT) teams at Cadence Child and Adolescent Therapy in Kirkland, Washington. She is a board-certified DBT clinician. Dr. Keller's areas of specialty with children, adolescents, and their families include emotion dysregulation, anxiety, depression, self-harm, suicidal thoughts and behavior, and parent training.

Foreword

I started off my career 40 years ago as a special-needs teacher, working with young children who were struggling to learn to read. They often came to me with significant frustration or hopelessness, having failed over and over again in their regular classrooms. They frequently posed behavioral challenges as well. I wish I had had this book when I first started teaching. It would have made me a far more effective teacher. Fortunately, providers now have *CBT Express* for their work with children and adolescents and their families.

Many children struggle with behavioral and mental health issues. When families bravely share a struggle with a professional, they need more than support. They need tools for change. Surprisingly, sometimes even a single intervention can make a significant difference in a family's functioning. But providers are often at a loss for what to do. They need help so they can better help children and their families.

The professionals to whom families reveal their difficulties work in a variety of settings: schools, primary care offices, clinics, or other hospital settings. Families frequently experience barriers to accessing evidence-based treatment, and providers are challenged with how to give families an effective intervention they can use right away. *CBT Express* offers specific, step-by-step interventions for providers and families. The authors' approach is unique in their ability to boil down theoretically sound interventions into doable steps for providers in different roles and professions. While a background in cognitive-behavioral therapy (CBT) is helpful, it's not essential: the stand-alone strategies are well described with case examples, worksheets, and illustrations. The text clearly describes what the professional can say and do.

Providers working with children and adolescents today need to impact symptoms in the often short period of time they have with families. Their interactions may take place in a few therapy sessions, a brief clinic consultation, a visit with a pediatrician or other health care provider, or a school counseling session between classes. Psychoeducation, used by many providers, generally is not, by itself, enough. Families need brief and effective strategies that they can start using immediately. The 10- to 15-minute interventions in this book include real-time practicing during the brief sessions with families. This practice is crucial and makes it far more likely that families will follow through and use these strategies at home.

Although many CBT books are available, *CBT Express* is truly different, focusing on quick and easy-to-implement CBT interventions to address symptoms while maintaining the theoretical basis and strong evidence base of CBT. This book offers a practical resource for providers in alternative settings, while also supplementing the toolkit of providers in more traditional therapy settings. By broadening the CBT expertise and knowledge of professionals interacting with youth, this book addresses the gap between patient–family needs and access to evidence-based treatments.

CBT Express uses a train metaphor to demonstrate the fast, "get right to it" intervention approach, while also following a clear track of CBT principles and evidence-based treatment interventions to reach the final destination: a reduction in symptoms, especially improvement in mood and behavior. The interventions are presented through an easy-to-understand framework so providers can quickly identify targets and introduce strategies to families. The strategies also build on one another and naturally build on those introduced previously.

Physicians, nurses, school counselors, therapists, and paraprofessionals often struggle with capitalizing on small periods of time with patients and families with mental and behavioral health needs. Many families disregard referrals to therapists. By the time other families get an appointment for traditional therapy, the crisis or opportunity to intervene may have passed. Other priorities may have emerged and symptoms can often go untreated. This book gives providers clear direction to begin addressing the mental health needs of families and offers concrete tools regardless of what past or future treatment might look like. By responding to families' concerns in the moment, the interventions in this book will help providers build trust with families and therefore increase engagement in future treatment.

The "What the Therapist Can Do" and "What the Therapist Can Say" sections in each chapter offer quick guides and sample language to keep interventions focused, effective, and short. Readers will enjoy the engaging dialogues and realistic examples used throughout the text. The HQ (Handy and Quick) Cards prompt families to use the interventions at home, while also priming families for future treatment by illustrating the connection between provider-introduced interventions and practices at home. *CBT Express* is an excellent investment for providers working with young patients who are looking to increase their impact on mental and behavioral health concerns. I think you'll find it both valuable and inspiring.

JUDITH S. BECK, PhD
Beck Institute for Cognitive Behavior Therapy
University of Pennsylvania

Contents

Purchasers of this book can download and print the HQ Cards
at *www.guilford.com/mcclure-forms* for personal use
or use with clients (see copyright page for details).

List of HQ CARDs

CHAPTER 4

CHAPTER 5

CHAPTER 6

CHAPTER 7

CHAPTER 8

Introduction to *CBT Express*

What?? Not Another CBT Techniques Book!: Why We Wrote *CBT Express*

When we were approached to write another book on cognitive-behavioral therapy (CBT) with youth, we immediately thought, "Do we really need *another* book on CBT with youth?" There are *so many* CBT texts available and we did not want to flood the market. We all decided that if we undertook this project, we wanted to do something *different*! Therefore, when we set out to write this book, we focused on the need for quick, easy-to-implement CBT interventions in the context of the expanding behavioral health care models.

Integrated behavioral health in pediatric primary care is emerging as a new frontier for CBT-oriented clinicians (Asarnow et al., 2015; Asarnow, Kolko, Miranda, & Kazak, 2017; Janicke, Fritz, & Rozensky, 2015). Behavioral health problems inundate pediatric practices and overburden pediatricians (Campo et al., 2005; Friedberg, Thordarson, Paternostro, Sullivan, & Tamas, 2014; Weitzman & Leventhal, 2006). While there is a surplus of children requiring behavioral health services, there is a corresponding shortage of skilled clinicians ready to care for them (Serrano, Cordes, Cubic, & Daub, 2018). The ability to deliver brief assessment and intervention is crucial. Expertise in brief CBT-based treatment methods would serve patients, providers, and clinics well.

As the behavioral health needs of children and adolescents continue to rise, there are numerous barriers to treatment for many children. A gap exists between mental health needs and access to evidence-based mental health treatment. To address this gap, we see more and more systems integrating mental health services into other settings to offer alternatives to the traditional outpatient psychotherapy model. Behavioral health therapy services are being provided in school settings and are integrated into primary care and specialty care clinics. These exciting innovations necessitate briefer interventions that can fit into shorter treatment sessions. The dynamic and shifting landscape of behavioral health care requires clinical flexibility. Several leading clinical child psychologists predict that clinicians will need to become comfortable intervening in sessions that are shorter than the traditional 50-minute hour (Asnarnow et al., 2015; Janicke et al., 2015). Finally, even when children and families present in traditional outpatient therapy settings, the length of treatment may only be a few visits, and thus every interaction needs to be focused and should include meaningful and effective interventions.

What *CBT Express* *Is* and *Is Not*

This book offers *express,* or efficient and effective, CBT interventions that can typically be implemented in 15 minutes or less. This express approach is like a train, efficient and fast, but also clearly traveling on a track (see Figure 1.1). Like the ties connected on a railroad track, the interventions and strategies presented in this book are connected to key CBT principles and proven evidence-based treatment interventions. Although different routes can be taken, the key features of CBT must be followed in order to reach the destination of symptom reduction. With a strong basis in CBT principles, the express interventions in this book offer providers a way to quickly identify meaningful points of intervention, teach and model effective strategies, and, most importantly, to then practice the strategy with the family in real time. Doing so not only facilitates the learning process but also increases family buy-in as family members immediately see an impact from the interventions and they develop hope for future improvements in symptoms.

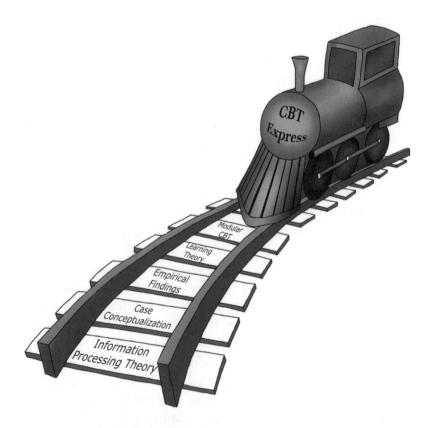

FIGURE 1.1. The *CBT Express* train.

Fortunately, the literature on CBT with children and adolescents is filled with many excellent textbooks that offer rich backgrounds in theory and research as well as practical applications (Flessner & Piacentini, 2017; Friedberg & McClure, 2015; Friedberg, McClure, & Hillwig-Garcia, 2009; Kendall, 2017; Manassis, 2009, 2012; Nangle et al., 2016; Sburlati et al., 2016; Weisz & Kazdin, 2017). Readers who are new to CBT or want a text that comprehensively reviews the theory/research should make the references just cited their "go-to" resources.

While all the procedures and practices are firmly rooted in the theoretical and empirical literature, this is not a textbook. Rather, *CBT Express* is a clinical toolkit. In *CBT Express*, we do not present a full discussion of the theoretical rationale and/or empirical support for any of the interventions. We offer very brief summaries of the foundational literature and suggest resources for further reading.

Additionally, there is little guidance on case conceptualization. We expect that readers who dig into this toolbox are already well schooled in the fundamentals of case conceptualization. If readers' case conceptualization skills need to be built from the ground up, they should metabolize the material contained in Friedberg and McClure (2015); Beck (2011); Kuyken, Padesky, and Dudley (2008); Persons (2008); and Manassis (2014). A list of user qualifications is presented in a go/no-go test in Figure 1.2.

CBT Express is designed to be a unique clinical tool. We offer practicing clinicians ready-to-use skills that can be delivered in approximately 15-minute segments of a session. The techniques are presented in their simplest, barest, and unplugged form. Interventions are described in sound-bite style to facilitate easy consumption.

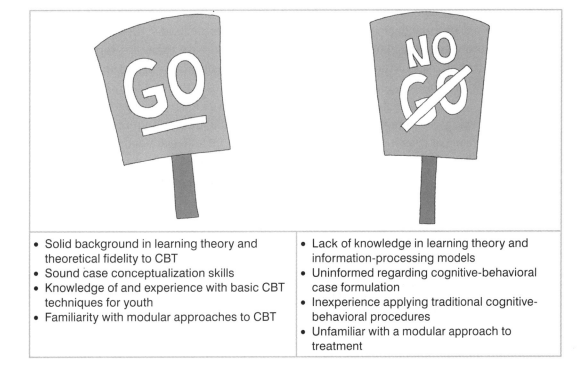

• Solid background in learning theory and theoretical fidelity to CBT • Sound case conceptualization skills • Knowledge of and experience with basic CBT techniques for youth • Familiarity with modular approaches to CBT	• Lack of knowledge in learning theory and information-processing models • Uninformed regarding cognitive-behavioral case formulation • Inexperience applying traditional cognitive-behavioral procedures • Unfamiliar with a modular approach to treatment

FIGURE 1.2. Go/no-go rules for using *CBT Express*.

Based on the conceptual scheme outlined in previous work (Friedberg et al., 2009; Friedberg, Gorman, Hollar-Wilt, Biuckians, & Murray, 2012), procedures are classified by their modular membership (psychoeducation, target monitoring, basic behavioral tasks, cognitive restructuring, and experiments/exposures). Modules represent the pistons of the *CBT Express* engine (see Figure 1.3). They make the therapy process go! An eclectic array of procedures is contained in each module. Although we do not include a full description of modular CBT, we do provide a brief description of these working parts as a reminder to readers.

Psychoeducation primes patients for therapy by teaching them about their presenting problems and the course of therapy. The information may be conveyed via verbal instruction, pamphlets, workbooks, books, games, music, video, and internet sites. Target monitoring locates treatment goals and grades progress. Formal symptom measures, indices of functional improvement, and user experience/patient satisfaction instruments may serve as target metrics. Basic behavioral tasks include procedures to modify patients' activities. Behavioral activation, relaxation, social skills, mindfulness, distress tolerance, and contingency contracting are examples of basic behavioral tasks. Cognitive restructuring involves simple and complex ways to help patients build better, more accurate, and productive interpretations of themselves, others, and their experiences. Self-instruction, problem solving, reattribution, tests of evidence, and decatastrophizing are cognitive restructuring tasks. The final module is experiments and exposure, where patients demonstrate the application of their coping skills while facing what they previously avoided. Touching contaminated surfaces without excessive washing, reading aloud in front of groups of peers, and completing a frustrating, demanding task without verbal or physical aggression are types of experiments and exposures.

This book offers interventions for providers to implement quickly, regardless of the setting. These interventions are designed for use across settings, and they are designed to be implemented by providers in various disciplines. Titles including therapist, provider, and clinician are used throughout the chapters' scripts, and case examples represent the various professional roles of those who will find these interventions useful in their work with children, adolescents, and families. Similarly, we recognize that the families with whom we work have a variety of relationships, and caregiver roles can vary. Therefore, some examples in the following chapters include cases that reference a specific parent (mother or father), while others make reference to a caregiver that could include extended family members. In order to protect the confidentiality of our patients, all of the case examples are fictionalized or disguised clinical accounts. They represent a combination of our many cases.

Structure of the Chapters

At the ends of Chapters 2–8, readers will find useful handouts and worksheets in the form of Handy and Quick (HQ) Cards. The HQ Cards are full of helpful information and reminders about *CBT Express* interventions and will help families recall what was covered during the visit. We have also included sample worksheets completed to illustrate the techniques. Providers can quickly reference and use these HQ Cards in real time with families, as they are organized by presenting concern. In addition, the HQ Cards then guide families in using the *Express* interventions at home.

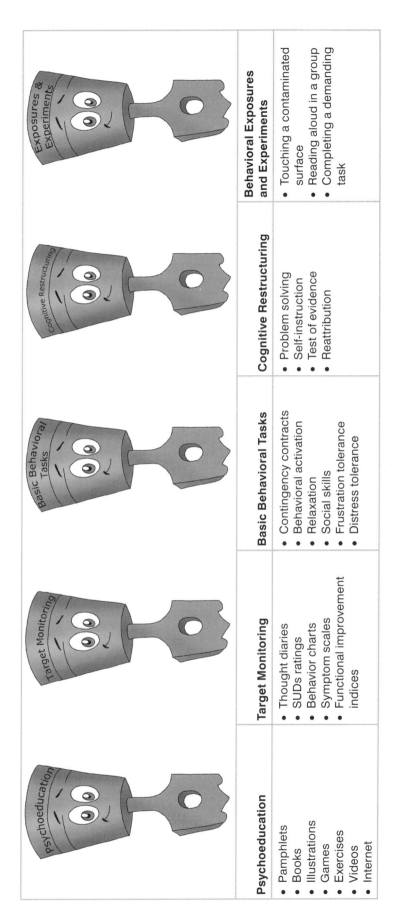

Psychoeducation	Target Monitoring	Basic Behavioral Tasks	Cognitive Restructuring	Behavioral Exposures and Experiments
• Pamphlets • Books • Illustrations • Games • Exercises • Videos • Internet	• Thought diaries • SUDs ratings • Behavior charts • Symptom scales • Functional improvement indices	• Contingency contracts • Behavioral activation • Relaxation • Social skills • Frustration tolerance • Distress tolerance	• Problem solving • Self-instruction • Test of evidence • Reattribution	• Touching a contaminated surface • Reading aloud in a group • Completing a demanding task

FIGURE 1.3. Pistons of the *CBT Express* engine.

Sample dialogues and scripts direct providers on how to efficiently introduce and move through the techniques in a meaningful way within 15 minutes. The "What the Therapist Can Say" and "What the Therapist Can Do" sections demonstrate how to keep the families focused on the interventions, even in the context of complex clinical pictures.

Chapter 2 offers guidance for identifying the treatment target, and Chapters 3 through 8 provide interventions for those targets once they are identified. Each intervention follows a rubric for easy reference and use by providers. The target age for the intervention, module, purpose, rationale, materials needed, and expected time for completion are all summarized at the start of each *Express* intervention to help providers choose the interventions quickly.

Readers can take the *CBT Express* to numerous settings and apply the techniques to a variety of presenting concerns and populations. We hope you enjoy the ride!

Locating the Treatment Target

Ready . . . Aim . . . Target!

What Is This Chapter About?

We include this chapter in *CBT Express* for an important reason. Even though this book is designed to provide you with innumerable clinical strategies, a critical first step is correctly identifying a treatment target. The procedures will fall flat if they are aimed at an incorrect mark. For instance, if you attempt to change an emotionally sanitized cognition with a handy and quick cognitive restructuring technique, young patients' mental sets are likely to stay the same and they may even complain they already understand their thinking is off, but the intervention does not help them to feel better.

Chapters 3 through 8 include sections that offer you a very basic conceptual framework for many *CBT Express* procedures. Functional analysis (FA) provides a context for the behavioral and cognitive procedures. Measurement-based care (MBC) is central to both good clinical care and future financial reimbursement. Incorporating MBC principles into your practice gives you feedback on how well treatment is going and is a form of continuous quality improvement (CQI). Moreover, it is extremely likely that most third-party payers will require measurement-based feedback to ensure their dollars are buying value-based services.

In sum, this chapter serves a threefold purpose. First, the material provides necessary conceptual roots for the *Express* procedures. Second, the chapter emphasizes the importance of identifying treatment targets and measuring progress toward goals. Third, readers are alerted to the likely necessity of practicing MBC in the context of behavioral health care reform.

Functional Analysis: Theoretical and Empirical Background

FA has a long tradition in developing an understanding of behavioral actions in cognitive-behavioral-spectrum approaches (Cone, 1997; Haynes, O'Brien, & Kaholokula, 2011; Kazdin,

2001; McLeod, Jensen-Doss, & Ollendick, 2013). FA's roots lie in operant and classical learning paradigms. Functional behavior simply means that the action is purposeful and goal oriented. Our behaviors and actions are directed toward increasing the likelihood of positive consequences or escaping adverse outcomes. Kazdin (2001) cogently explained, "the goal of functional analysis is to identify the conditions that control the occurrence and maintenance of behavior" (p. 103).

The use of FA provides several advantages for clinicians (Kazdin, 2001). First, when you specify the cues and consequences of the problem behavior, the parameters surrounding the difficulty become more apparent. Second, actions are better understood by viewing them within the context in which they took place. Third, children's self-control is optimized. More specifically, when triggers and contingent outcomes are identified, young people can be taught skills to cope with stressors and seek productive actions.

In sum, FA maps out the behavior. Completing an FA helps you quickly identify the dynamic context in which actions exist and the factors that influence their frequency, intensity, and duration.

Alphabet City:
The ABC's of Functional Analysis

FA takes shape through the ABC model. "A" refers to *antecedents*, which are cues that provoke the behavior. A's could be stimuli that directly lead to the behavior such as being bullied, taking a test, or the breakup of a relationship. Additionally, surrounding or background conditions that set the stage for the behavior are also A's. Examples include the presence of certain people, the time of day, or the noise level in the room. Finally, internal stimuli can prompt children's actions. These internal cues could be increased heart rate, muscle tension, and negative affective experiences.

B's refer to target *behaviors*, or what we like to call "the usual suspects." These behaviors are the problem behaviors or actions that clinicians seek to change. It is very important to be as precise as possible when identifying B's. Targeting vague B's can cause therapeutic interventions to misfire. Considerable effort is required to pin down these usual suspects. Caregivers, teachers, and young patients themselves often describe the usual suspects in broad strokes. For example, adults may complain about young people having bad attitudes or not listening, or patients may describe feeling "weird," which requires the therapist to concretize the problem in specific terms.

HQ Card 2.1 (p. 15) guides you in pinning down the "usual behavioral suspect" shrouded in the child's or caregiver's description of the general complaint. In the left-hand column, labeled "the usual suspect," the child's presenting problem is shown as a vaguely constructed issue (e.g., school is boring). On the right side, simple queries are suggested to help you operationally define treatment targets.

C's are *consequences* that make the B's more or less likely to recur. In general, C's are classified as reinforcers or punishers. Reinforcers may either be positive or negative. Many practitioners get unnecessarily confused about negative reinforcement. Just keep in mind a few simple points. Both positive reinforcement and negative reinforcement serve to *increase* the function of the behavior. However, positive reinforcement involves adding (+) something pleasant (+) to increase the behavior. On the other hand, negative reinforcement is subtracting or removing (–) something negative (–) to increase behavior.

Rewards earn their value through the eye of the beholder. Remember, rewards carry power only if children prize them. Therefore, you will need to work to find the reinforcement value of different rewards. HQ Card 2.2 (p. 16) gives you some questions to ask caregivers and children to find the desired rewards.

The most typical consequences that decrease frequency of behavior are response cost and punishment procedures. Time-out and removal of rewards and privileges are typical response cost procedures.

HQ Card 2.3 (p. 17) serves as a handy reminder about positive reinforcement, negative reinforcement, and response cost.

The ABC rubric forms the architecture of FA. Precisely locating the A's and C's yields a clinical road map. HQ Card 2.4 (p. 18) gives you specific questions to find the A's and C's as you navigate through Alphabet City. To find the correct place on A Street, check out the left column of the card. Questions on the right side track down the correct spot on C Street.

After you and your patients specify the A and C routes to children's behaviors (B), you are ready design a personalized map to Alphabet City for your patient. Figures 2.1 and 2.2 show you the way.

In Figure 2.1, Jody's compliant behavior (B) is cued by an effective command (A) (e.g., "Jody, please come down to dinner."). In turn, Jody's compliant behavior is followed by contingent positive reinforcement (e.g., "Because you did what I said, you may choose dessert tonight."). Compliance is established by clear commands and positive reinforcement.

Figure 2.2 maps out Andre's avoidant behavior. Andre experiences antecedent triggers (A) (e.g., seeing announcement, feeling anxious). He then avoids the team meeting and makes a catastrophic prediction (e.g., "Everyone will think I am a wannabe."). His escape behavior is negatively reinforced by relief from his anxiety. His avoidance is maintained through the temporary relief of his anxiety.

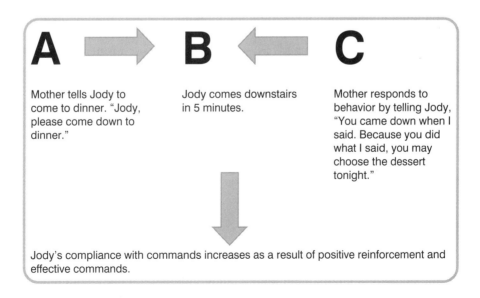

FIGURE 2.1. Sample map for Jody's Alphabet City.

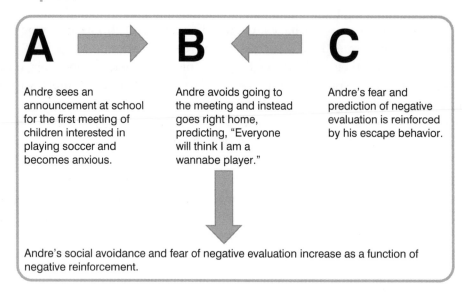

FIGURE 2.2. Sample Map for Andre's Alphabet City.

Common Interventions Based on Functional Analysis

Giving good commands or instructions, doling out praise and rewards, removing privileges and rewards, and conducting effective time-outs are common procedures born out of functional analyses. You can find specific applications of these interventions in Chapter 3 (on noncompliance). In this section, we provide you with some basic broad-spectrum rubrics.

Giving Good Commands

Giving good commands is a first step toward teaching children to behave according to reasonable expectations. In order to help children learn to comply, you will need to coach parents, teachers, and other caregivers about how to give effective requests. FA shows you the way!

We refer to making commands as "calling signals." The tips in HQ Card 2.5 (p. 19) are based on fundamental concepts in FA. First, you must ensure the caregiver captures the child's attention (e.g., makes eye contact). Second, caregivers should make clear, polite, and calm commands. Third, requests should not include "let's" (e.g., "Let's clean up the dishes"), "we" (e.g., "We need to get our shoes on"), or "why" (e.g., "Why don't you get started on your chores") statements. Rather, the calling signals are specific and direct ("I need you to put the dishes in the dishwasher before going outside"; "Put your shoes on now, please"; "It is time to pick up your dirty clothes."). Finally, good signal callers do not flood children with multiple and/or unnecessary commands. Caregivers need to be picky about the battles they elect to fight.

Delivering Praise and Rewards

Positive reinforcement is the best way to build productive behavior. However, delivering praise and rewards is not as easy as it may appear. Based on extensive research on learning theory, several authors (Chorpita & Weisz, 2009; Nangle, Hansen, Grover, Kingery, & Suveg, 2016) have identified the nuggets of effective praise and reinforcement.

HQ Card 2.6 (p. 20), an aid for parents and clinicians, lists basic strategies for effective praise statements. First, good praise is specific (e.g., "You got all your homework done tonight!") rather than vague (e.g., "Good going"). The second point to communicate to parents is that they do not have to praise every behavior. Praise should be heaped upon behaviors that reflect new learning. Parents and caregivers need to spot behaviors they want to increase that are occurring at a low frequency or are just beginning to emerge. Those behaviors should be the targets of praise and rewards.

Immediate rewards are preferred over delayed consequences. This is especially true for impulsive children and those young people who find it difficult to delay gratification. Praise and rewards should be linked to the behavior you are seeking to increase. Caregivers' reward cupboards should be fully stocked with a variety of positive reinforcers that range in magnitude. Finally, the type and magnitude of the reward should match children's behavioral achievements (e.g., small accomplishment = small reward; big accomplishment = big reward).

Removing Rewards and Privileges

Removing rewards and privileges is a response cost procedure. When a child misbehaves, he or she has to pay a cost. Typically, the penalty involves taking away a valued reward or privilege. Various sources offer fundamentals for removing rewards and privileges (Chorpita & Weisz, 2009; Kazdin, 2008).

HQ Card 2.7 (p. 21) gives parents helpful reminders about removing rewards and privileges. First, like presenting rewards and privileges, withdrawing them needs to be explicitly linked to children's behaviors (e.g. "Because you hit your sister when you were both playing with the iPad, you may not play with it tonight."). Second, the type of reward or privilege removed and the length it is withdrawn should match the child's misbehavior. Regardless of the child's impropriety, rewards and privileges should not be removed for long periods of time. If children are forced to live without something for even a week, they will learn to live without it, making the behavioral management strategy less effective. Finally, Kazdin (2008) recommends a minimum ratio of five reinforcing statements/rewards to any one response cost procedure.

Conducting Effective Time-Outs

Time-out is another response cost procedure. Simply, time-out refers to removing the child from a reinforcing situation as a penalty for misbehavior. As with other procedures, readers are referred to sources that more fully describe these behavior management strategies (Chorpita & Daleiden, 2009; Drayton et al., 2012; Kazdin, 2008).

HQ Card 2.8 (p. 22) offers pointers for implementing time-out. First, time-out should be done immediately following the undesirable behavior. Experts agree that the commands to go to time-out should be brief and to the point. Chorpita and Weisz (2009) suggest a handy rudiment ("10 for 10") where the command is given in 10 seconds with 10 words. Time-out begins when the child is sitting down and quiet. Short time-outs are preferable to long ones. Many parenting professionals agree that time-outs should be no more than 1 minute per age of the child (e.g., 4-year-old child = 4-minute time-out), although this is not a rigid rule. For many children who are on the older end of the 2–11 range, a shorter time-out is both effective and more manageable for caregivers. Finally, after time-out ends, parents and caretakers need to look for opportunities to praise the child for desirable alternate behaviors.

Hey, UMP!: Unique Mental Parcels

As cognitive-behavioral therapists readily recognize, automatic thoughts (ATs) drive most children's experiences. However, not all thoughts are created equal. Some thoughts are benign and not emotionally painful. Other beliefs carry an emotional wallop. As a clinician working on the *CBT Express*, you will want to quickly and efficiently identify the AT with the highest affective payload. In order to do this, you will need to identify the unique mental parcels (UMPs). This section helps you recognize which thoughts go with different distressing feelings.

Theoretical and Empirical Background

The content-specificity hypothesis (CSH) is supported by much bench or laboratory science investigating cognitive products accompanying particular emotional states (Cho & Telch, 2005; Ghahramanlou-Holloway, Wenzel, Lou, & Beck, 2007; Lamberton & Oei, 2008; Schniering & Rapee, 2002). Interested readers are referred to Beck (1976) as well as Friedberg and McClure (2015) for greater coverage on this topic.

The CSH allows clinicians to identify emotionally charged thoughts. Additionally, the CSH is a useful way to separate multiple thoughts and feelings. For example, in clinical practice, children and adolescents often experience multiple feelings and thoughts regarding the same situation. Knowing what thoughts go with which emotions allows clinicians to sort out the specific connections.

According to the CSH, depression is characterized by themes of loss, deprivation, and defeat. Depression is accompanied by a negative view of the self (e.g., "I'm a loser"), negative view of others and one's experiences (e.g., "Others are out to get me"), and negative view of the future (e.g., "Things will never get better"). Anxiety's core theme is danger or threat. When children experience danger, they overestimate the probability and magnitude of the danger, neglect rescue factors, and often ignore coping resources. As an alert reader, you may recognize overestimation of the magnitude of danger as catastrophizing. Social anxiety carries catastrophic content that emphasizes the fear of negative evaluation. Panic involves the catastrophic misinterpretation of normal bodily sensations.

When children experience anger, they focus critical attention on others rather than themselves. The specific content centers on making hostile attributions about other people's behaviors, which includes labeling the other person, believing someone has ruptured one's own privately held rules, and inaccurately perceiving unwanted outcomes as unfair. HQ Card 2.9 (p. 23) presents a clinician's pocket guide to the CSH.

HQ Card 2.10 (p. 24) is a practitioner's guide to identifying meaningful cognitions. "I Spy" questions are provided to help you precisely isolate the unique cognitive content associated with different moods. The "I Spy" queries are an illustrative but not exhaustive list. So feel free to modify them as long as you stay true to the goal of digging for the various themes (e.g., danger, loss, violation).

Measurement-Based Care

In the new era of behavioral health care reform, quality counts (Friedberg & Rozbruch, 2016). When writing about reimbursement issues for psychotherapy many years ago, Barker

(1983) stated, "No one will be willing to continually pay large sums of money for anything unless they are sure of its worth" (p. 76). This prophetic statement remains quite true more than 30 years later. Value for the behavioral health care dollar is the new watchword. Providers who bring good outcomes to patients' problems will receive payment premiums (Bickman, 2008; Kirch & Ast, 2017; Unutzer et al., 2012).

Clinicians and patients profit from ongoing feedback about treatment progress (Scott & Lewis, 2015). When patients do better during and after the course of treatment, patients and providers benefit. In a broader sense, better service provision raises public confidence in child psychotherapy. Consequently, more referrals are generated and reimbursement rates are likely to increase. Finally, greater provision of quality care crowds "lemons" out of the behavioral health care marketplace.

Friedberg (2015) discussed the problem of "lemons" in psychotherapy. A lemon is a poor product or service that is dissatisfying to consumers (Akerof, 1970). Naturally, people do not pay premium prices for bad services. When lemons abound in a market, poor-quality services and product persist, and overall value for similar services declines. Friedberg (2015) noted that in these circumstances, "everything has equal value and is valued at the lowest price" (p. 339). Therefore, MBC is a way to monitor quality and demonstrate that your services are peaches rather than lemons.

MBC has gained a great deal of appeal in helping to improve clinical work with children and adolescents. Simply put, MBC refers to the process of regularly and repeatedly collecting patient outcomes over time to assess progress (Bickman, 2008; Bickman, Kelley, Breda, de Andrade, & Riemer, 2011). MBC is related to increased treatment progress (Lambert et al., 2002). Moreover, in young patients, MBC was associated with a quicker rate of improvement (Bickman et al., 2011). In their review, Scott and Lewis (2015) summarized the findings of multiple studies showing that MBC resulted in better decision making and judgments by clinicians.

MBC allows for both clinicians and patients to evaluate the return on their investment. Simply, these metrics shed light on what is working in treatment. Regular treatment monitoring facilitates necessary adjustments during the treatment process. It informs practitioners on when to stay the treatment course and when to make corrections. Further, MBC lets clinicians know what type of corrections could be made if they are indicated.

Tracking Numbers

If you have ever ordered something online or used a parcel delivery service, you know about tracking numbers. A tracking number serves to monitor the process from shipment to receipt. In this way, if the shipment gets derailed or lost, there is a way to identify or correct it. This is exactly what we as CBT therapists do to monitor treatment progress. In order to effectively and efficiently deliver a proper dose of *CBT Express*, therapists need to employ meaningful metrics to evaluate progress toward goals.

There are numerous ways for you to assess treatment outcome. These methods could reflect functional improvements, symptom reductions, and/or user experiences (Scott & Lewis, 2015). Additionally, depending on the circumstances of your practice, these methods could be standardized measures or individually constructed. Regardless of what type of measure you elect to employ, these tools should be simple, quick, and relevant to clinical concerns. Simply, value is multiply determined by a combination of measurement-based instruments.

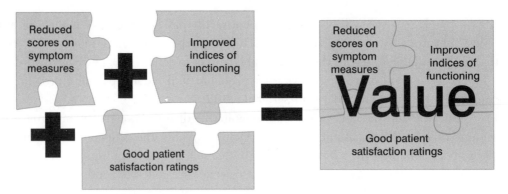

FIGURE 2.3. Assessing treatment outcomes.

Figure 2.3 illustrates the point. Accordingly, we recommend that clinicians employ diverse ways to demonstrate the value-added benefits of the services they provide.

Measures of functional improvement are personalized metrics designed to track improvement in individual patients' functioning. These functional indices might involve recording number of missed school days, visits to the school nurse, lowered medication dosages, and so on. HQ Card 2.11 (p. 25) lists several handy examples of functional improvement metrics. It should be noted that functional improvements are quite compelling to payers and patients alike. However, changes in functional outcomes can be hard to come by. Perhaps this is the reason they are so compelling.

Reductions on objective symptom measures are commonly used to track progress. There are many choices for objective symptom inventories. Friedberg et al. (2009) listed frequently selected scales that are both copyrighted and in the public domain. In a very comprehensive review, Beidas et al. (2015) outlined free, low-cost, valid, and reliable measures that are especially attractive to agencies, clinics, and practitioners with lean budgets.

User Experience

In addition to tracking numbers, user experience measures are helpful for evaluating care. User experience instruments tap patients' and families' perception of treatment and satisfaction with their services. Scott and Lewis (2015) noted that treatment alliance measures are essentially user experience measures. Finally, Miller (2015) argued that third-party payers pay special attention to patient satisfaction ratings.

Conclusion

Armed with an understanding of FA, the CSF, and MBC, you are ready to continue on the *CBT Express*. The following chapters will build upon these principles and offer specific applications of effective CBT interventions for express implementation in a variety of settings. HQ Cards (Handy and Quick worksheets and handouts) found at the ends of the chapters will serve as cues and reminders for families and clinicians when implementing the interventions at home, at school, or in a clinic or hospital setting.

Sample Questions to Pin Down the Usual Suspects

The usual suspect	Questions to capture the usual suspect
School is too boring for me.	• What things about school are boring? • What things are interesting? • How can you tell the difference? • If school was not so boring, what would be different? • How do you react when you are stuck in boring school all day? • How do you let other people know you are bored?
He doesn't listen.	• What does he do when he doesn't listen? • How does he act? • How do you know he is not listening? • How can you know when he is listening?
I feel weird.	• What do you do when you feel weird? • How would others know you feel weird? • What goes through your mind when you feel weird?

Digging for Reinforcers

What activities does _____ do a lot?

What does _____ do for fun?

What is an uplift for _____?

What brightens _____ mood?

What makes _____ feel good?

What makes _____ feel better?

What does _____ value?

What is _____ willing to work for?

What does _____ enjoy?

_____

From *CBT Express* by Jessica M. McClure, Robert D. Friedberg, Micaela A. Thordarson, and Marisa Keller. Copyright © 2019 The Guilford Press. Permission to photocopy this HQ Card is granted to purchasers of this book for personal use or use with clients (see copyright page for details). Purchasers can download additional copies of this HQ Card (see the box at the end of the table of contents).

Reminders about Positive Reinforcement, Negative Reinforcement, and Response Cost

Positive Reinforcement	Something PLEASANT OR DESIRABLE (+) is ADDED and behavior subsequently INCREASES.

- Sammy completes his homework and his father plays a special computer game with him. Subsequently, his homework compliance increases.
- This is reinforcement because the effect of the procedure is to INCREASE behavior.
- It is positive because something PLEASANT is ADDED.

Negative Reinforcement	Something UNPLEASANT OR UNDESIRABLE is REMOVED and behavior subsequently INCREASES.

- Daniela finds her choir teacher's critical comments to be aversive. Subsequently, she continues to skip choir practice.
- This process is reinforcement because Daniela's escape and avoidance behavior INCREASES.
- It is negative because the UNPLEASANT stimulus is SUBTRACTED OR REMOVED.

Response Cost	Misbehavior results in a child receiving a penalty such as REMOVING a reward or privilege. The effect is a DECREASE in the frequency of the misbehavior recurring.

- Matilda purposefully breaks several of her sister's crayons when they are coloring. Her mother takes the rest of the crayons away from her for the remainder of the day. Subsequently, Matilda plays with her sister without damaging her things in the future.
- It is a response cost because the misbehavior causes her to pay a cost.

Specifying the ABC's

A?	B?	C?
What words do you use when you make requests and commands? How do you tell people to do something? When do you make commands/requests? What happens just before? What goes through your mind right before _____? What feelings do you have before _____? Who is around when you _____?		What happens after? What follows _____ behavior? How do you let _____ know you approve/disapprove of what he/she does? What do you get out of _____? What does _____ give you?

Calling Signals: Giving Effective Commands

✓ Make eye contact.

✓ Be polite and calm.

✓ Stay clear and to the point.

✓ Avoid "why," "let's," and/or "we" commands.

✓ Remain choosy about the time when you make a request.

✓ Be picky about the number and types of commands and requests you make.

LESS IS ALWAYS MORE.

Tips for Giving Effective Praise

✓ Good praise is specific.

"You rocked that math test. Your studying really paid off!" instead of "Nice work."

✓ Do not praise every behavior or accomplishment. You should praise behavior that is new and age-appropriate for your child.

✓ These statements should follow the desired behavior as soon as possible.

✓ Be enthusiastic with praise.

✓ Consider coupling the praise with a hug or pat on the back if the young person values physical affection.

IT IS IMPORTANT TO BE ON THE LOOKOUT FOR TIMES WHEN CHILDREN ARE BEHAVING WELL SO PRAISE CAN BE DELIVERED FREQUENTLY.

Tips for Removing Rewards and Privileges

✓ Tie the penalty to the child's misbehavior.

"Because you did not feed the dog when I asked you, you will lose 10 minutes of screen time tonight."

✓ Match the value of the reward or privilege to the degree of misbehavior.

✓ Rely on removing a reward or privilege for shorter periods of time.

✓ Remember to look for instances of desirable behavior and balance every response cost with about five positive reinforcements (5-to-1 ratio).

Tips for Giving Time-Outs

✓ Time-outs should be delivered immediately after the misbehavior.

✓ Explanation for going to time-out should be brief and to the point.

  "Because you hit your brother, you need to go to time-out."

✓ Time-out begins when the child is sitting still and quiet.

✓ Short time-outs are just as effective as longer time-outs.

✓ Look for opportunities to praise the child for desirable behavior after leaving time-out.

Clinicians' Guide
to the Content-Specificity Hypothesis

Mood	Content: You have located a hot thought if it transparently communicates . . .
Depression	• Negative view of the self • Negative view of others and one's experiences • Negative view of the future
Anger	• Hostile attributional bias • Sense of unfairness • Labeling the other person • Violation of personal rules
Anxiety	• Overestimation of the magnitude of the danger • Overestimation of the probability of the danger • Neglect of rescue factors • Ignoring coping resources
Social anxiety	• Fear of negative evaluation
Panic	• Catastrophic misinterpretation of normal bodily sensations

I Spy the UMP

Mood	Sample "I Spy" Questions
Depression	• What negative judgments are you making?
	• What are you saying to yourself that beats you up?
	• In what ways are you putting yourself down?
	• What is your inner critic saying?
	• What negative things about yourself are bouncing around inside your head?
	• What gloomy tweets are popping up?
	• How much confidence do you have that things will work out for you?
	• How much do you FOMO (Fear of Missing Out)?
	• What do you see yourself as having lost?
	• What things do you not see as possible for you?
Anxiety	• What is the danger?
	• What is the risk?
	• What is the disaster?
	• What is the threat?
	• What horrible things are you expecting?
	• What terrible things are you guessing will happen?
	• What is overwhelming?
	• What does your mind's eye tell you about your ability to cope?
Anger	• What rules of yours are other people breaking?
	• What do you call someone who breaks your rules?
	• How fair do you see this to be?

Functional Outcome Metrics

- Lowered medication dosages

- Fewer school suspensions

- Fewer visits to the school nurse

- Reduced number of emergency room visits

- Decreased frequency of cutting

- Reduced number of fights

- Negative findings on drug urinalysis

Noncompliance

"He never listens."

"I can't get her to do anything unless she wants to do it."

"Her behavior—I don't know what to say, she's just bad."

We've all heard these familiar complaints from parents, either when parents are asked about their child's behavior or when the concerns are spontaneously raised by families seeking assistance for other problems.

Parents may express frustration in different ways, but the underlying message is often the same: behavioral difficulties are a primary concern for caregivers. Parents struggle with getting children and teens to do what they want them to do. They may use words or phrases such as *defiant, stubborn, bad, strong-willed,* or *won't listen.* At the core of all these comments is a desire for their children to do more of something (homework, using polite words, chores) or less of something (talking back, yelling, hitting, arguing).

These complaints are rooted in parents' desire to increase the child's compliance and decrease noncompliance with instructions or tasks. The reasons for a child's noncompliance are often far-ranging, and much time can be spent assessing when the noncompliance started, when it is better or worse, and possible triggers for noncompliance. Remember, we presented a simple rubric called Alphabet City in Chapter 2 to help you *quickly* map out children's behavioral difficulties.

Further, during treatment for other conditions, such as anxiety or depression, questions about behavior management often arise and could be addressed with some of the following strategies without derailing the primary treatment focus. The interventions in this chapter are based on evidence-based strategies for behavioral symptoms and are designed for *Express* implementation in most settings, regardless of whether compliance is the primary presenting problem or secondary to another presenting concern.

Brief Statement Regarding Evidence-Based Treatment

Externalizing behavior problems are one of the most common reasons parents seek treatment for their youngsters (Nock, Kazdin, Hiripi, & Kessler, 2007; Wolff & Ollendick, 2010). These behavior problems have been described as noncompliance, oppositionality, defiance, disruptive behavior, and externalizing behavior. There is a substantial body of research demonstrating that effective interventions exist for noncompliance in children and adolescents, yet no single approach has clearly emerged as "best" (Eyberg, Nelson, & Boggs, 2008).

However, the evidence-based treatments for noncompliance share significant commonalities that can be distilled into key components for effective treatment (Chorpita, Daleiden, & Weisz, 2005). To begin with, all are behavioral, cognitive-behavioral, and/or family systems based, and most include a significant parent component (Eyberg et al., 2008; McCart & Sheidow, 2016).

Parent training is considered first-line treatment for disruptive behavior in young children and a child-training component may be a beneficial addition for adolescents (Eyberg et al., 2008). Some of the most common interventions with strong empirical support include the Coping Power program (Lochman & Wells, 2004; Lochman et al., 2011), problem-solving skills training + parent management training (Kazdin, 2010; Lochman, Powell, Boxmeyer, & Jimenez-Camargo, 2011), Parent Management Training—Oregon model (PMTO; Patterson, Reid, Jones, & Conger, 1975), Helping the Noncompliant Child (HNC; Forehand & McMahon, 1981), the Incredible Years (IY; Webster-Stratton & Reid, 2003), multisystemic therapy (MST; Henggeler & Lee, 2003), and Parent–Child Interaction Therapy (PCIT; Brinkmeyer & Eyberg, 2003). Several meta-analyses support the effectiveness of CBT-based programs for the prevention and treatment of disruptive behavior (Lochman et al., 2011; Robinson, Smith, & Miller, 1999; Sukhodolsky, Kassinove, & Gorman, 2004). In short, there is a robust literature base supporting the effectiveness of CBT for noncompliance.

Parent training components share common elements that appear to be critical ingredients: psychoeducation about behavioral principles, increasing praise and positive interactions, ignoring minor disruptive behaviors, giving clear directions, and following through with consequences (Brinkmeyer & Eyberg, 2003; Forehand & McMahon, 1981; Patterson et al., 1975; Webster-Stratton & Reid, 2003). These are the same core components you will find in the *Express* strategies below.

Presenting Concerns and Symptoms

Therapists are like language interpreters, working with families to translate descriptions of their concerns with their children and transform them into clear behavioral goals. When you have little time with families, this can be challenging. Vague statements such as "He won't listen" or "She's just bad" need to be broken down into what exactly the parents mean. We find one of the quickest and most effect ways to do so is to ask parents what they would like the child to do differently that he or she is not doing now, and for the caregiver to give an example of when that happened recently (e.g., "today" or "this week").

By keeping families focused on the specific behaviors they would like to see change, providers can keep the momentum of treatment going and utilize the short time they have with families for intervention. It can be a balancing act for providers to have families feel heard and understood while also allotting enough time to intervene and have an impact on the symptoms causing the family distress. Simply offering empathy and active listening will help families feel heard and connected to the provider, but it will not lead to new skills in behavior management or much change in the targeted behaviors. Thus, therapists have to be skilled in incorporating active listening and demonstrating empathy while introducing, modeling, and practicing behavioral interventions with the family given time limitations that may exist. Chapter 2 outlined the importance of FA and the ABC model. The interventions below build on this approach to help therapists quickly identify what behaviors are impacting the family interactions, identify possible solutions, and work with the family to start an *Express* intervention.

Interventions

Take the following example of a family being seen in family therapy for Trace's significant separation anxiety and school refusal. During a session outlining exposures for anxiety symptoms, Trace's mom brought up an inability to get Trace to follow basic directions, even for tasks unrelated to school attendance.

> THERAPIST: We have been working on anxiety management techniques and the exposure hierarchy we created a few sessions ago, but when we set today's session agenda, you indicated you wanted to work on Trace's overall compliance with directions you give him.

> MOM: That's right. He never listens, and I always have to tell him the same thing over and over again. He is on his own schedule and only does things when he feels like it. I am tired of him ignoring me and just spending all weekend playing video games instead of helping out around the house or at the very least cleaning up after himself. I am constantly telling him to get his room picked up, but it is still a disaster.

> THERAPIST: It sounds like it is very frustrating when Trace doesn't do what you expect of him, and it also sounds like this has been an ongoing problem.

> MOM: Oh yes, he never really listens.

> THERAPIST: Why don't we start with what the expectations are and then figure out how to get Trace to meet your expectations?

> TRACE: I will tell you what the expectations are—she wants me to do everything around the house. She is never satisfied. It is constant nagging about cleaning and more cleaning. I can't help it if she is a neat freak. She wants me to do like 10 chores every day, and that doesn't leave me any time to relax or hang out.

> MOM: I don't expect it to be perfect, but I don't think you picking your underwear up off the bathroom floor is too much to ask.

> THERAPIST: What if we came up with just three things that Trace had to do every weekend? Would that be reasonable?

> TRACE: If you can keep her to three things, that would be a miracle.

> THERAPIST: So you would be OK with that?

> TRACE: Yeah, sure.

> THERAPIST: OK, and what about you, Mom? Does that sound reasonable?

> MOM: Sure, if he really does them.

THERAPIST: OK, so we all agree there will be three things that are expected as far as chores/cleanup for now. Trace, what are your guesses about what three things your mom will want?

TRACE: Ugh, I am sure she will say, "Clean room." She always says that like every day.

MOM: That would be amazing!

As a therapist, it might be tempting to now move on to the other two chores to be identified, especially if you are short on time. However, it is important to help the family clearly define the former chore first and ensure it is doable, or else at the next visit you are likely to hear, "It didn't work." Specifically, the therapist needs to work with the family to define what it means to have a "clean room," how often Trace will be expected to get his room back to this baseline, and how Trace will remember or be reminded of this responsibility. Estimating the time it will take to do this chore will be important, since part of Trace's frustration with chores is that he feels he spends "a ton" of time on chores and has little free time as a result. The challenge for the therapist is to identify these specifics in a quick and collaborative manner so the remaining time with the family can be spent on other interventions.

THERAPIST: OK, it sounds like you both agree with "clean room" as one of the chores, but we need to make sure everyone is on the same page with what a clean room means before we move on to figuring out what the other two chores will be.

MOM: No clothes on the floor! Clean clothes put away and dirty clothes in the hamper.

THERAPIST: Trace, how long do you think it will take you each weekend to pick up any clothes on the floor and either put them in your dresser, hang them up in your closet, or put them in the hamper if they are dirty?

TRACE: It depends. (*Rolls his eyes.*)

THERAPIST: True—what are you thinking it depends on?

TRACE: Well, if there is a clean basket of laundry to put away, that would take like 10 minutes just to put those close away. And then if I had practice and my basketball uniform was dirty, I would have to pick that up, plus my school clothes and whatever I wore to bed the night before.

THERAPIST: OK. How long to put your dirty basketball and school clothes in the hamper?

TRACE: (*grinning*) All right, I see where you are going with this. Sure, that would be quick—but all the other stuff added together is still a ton of my free time.

THERAPIST: Just humor me a bit longer. How many seconds or minutes to put those things in the hamper?

TRACE: Honestly, probably less than a minute.

THERAPIST: OK, and lastly you said the clothes you wore to bed. Do you usually wear those more than one night?

TRACE: Yeah.

THERAPIST: How long to put those away?

TRACE: I keep those in my dresser drawer. I don't know, I guess less than a minute too.

THERAPIST: OK, so we are up to a max of 12 minutes if it is a day you have a clean basket of laundry. Earlier we mapped out that your typical weekend includes a basketball game, homework, and youth group at church. Basketball is typically in the morning, and youth group at night, so from about noon to 6 you have free time and time for homework. You also mentioned you typically have 1 hour of homework over the weekend. With those activities and the 12 minutes that goes to cleaning up your room, how much time is left?

TRACE: OK, that sounds like a lot of time because it is almost 5 hours, but that is only one of the three chores.

THERAPIST: True, let's see what we can work out for those other two chores and see where we are.

(The therapist works with the family using the same process for the other two chores, and then develops a strategy with the family for following through with the plan.)

This discussion about chores could easily take an entire 45-minute session, but by staying focused on the specific details, the therapist and family were able to work through the entire process in a few minutes. If the time spent on the second and third chore is about the same length as that in the dialogue above, all three chores would be identified, outlined, and a plan devised in less than 10 minutes, and treatment could return to focusing on the primary concern of anxiety and school refusal.

The following sections of this chapter provide *Express* behavioral interventions for increasing compliance and improving motivation. The sample dialogues or scripts for introducing and practicing these strategies with families, as well as handouts and worksheets, will assist the reader in using these interventions with the children and families with whom they work.

Parenting Blocks for Modifying Behavior

Ages: Parents of children of all ages.

Module: Basic Behavioral Tasks.

Purpose: Increase parents' understanding and use of strategies for modifying behaviors.

Rationale: The basics of behavior modification will be helpful for parents trying to improve a number of behaviors in their child. By teaching the basics early in treatment, providers can help parents generalize behavioral interventions to numerous targets.

Materials: HQ Card 3.1, Building Blocks (p. 44), or four small wooden blocks labeled like the HQ Card 3.1 pictures.

Expected time needed: 5–10 minutes.

Parenting Blocks for Modifying Behavior assists with *Express* application of basic behavioral principles to the most common behavioral concerns you are likely to encounter when working with families. Whether parents have concerns about homework completion, chores, lack of follow-through, or low motivation, some basic behavioral strategies are key. The

Parenting Blocks provide quick visual cues for teaching and prompting caregivers to use specific behavioral interventions. They can easily be integrated into other *Express* interventions to prompt parents to use a behavioral technique in the midst of another intervention.

Praise

When asked, parents state they praise their children for good behavior. What therapists must attend to is the type and frequency of the praise. Upon further assessment or when observing parent–child interactions in sessions, it is often clear that parents' praise is vague and infrequent compared to the frequency of redirection or negative comments about behavior. Helping parents understand that any attention to a behavior is likely to increase the frequency of that behavior and giving them the tools to provide specific and frequent praise can assist in modifying many problematic patterns. The Tell, Show, Rehearse, Review, and Repeat intervention presented later in this chapter (pp. 33–35) is an excellent *Express* strategy for increasing caregiver use of effective praise and can be paired with the *Praise* parenting block.

Differential Attention

When working with parents on praise and attending to good behavior, the issue often arises that some negative behaviors need redirected. Teaching parents to provide differential attention can assist in getting buy-in from parents, as well as help parents understand the power of attention and ways they may be inadvertently reinforcing undesirable behaviors in their children.

Effective Directions

We all do it: we use questions as a way to be polite (e.g., "Can you get the door?"; "Will you please pass the salt?"; "Can you tell me what time it is?"). This habit is so ingrained we often are not aware we are posing these as questions. Parents often apply this same linguistic pattern with their children (e.g., "Can you pick up your shoes?"; "Will you please set the table?"; "Can you tell me what you have for homework?"). This can lead to a struggle because when asked these questions, children believe they have a choice and will respond with "no." They are not interpreting the questions as a polite instruction. They make their choice ("no") and then are reprimanded for it, which often results in frustration on the part of the child and increased parent–child conflict. We teach parents to give simple, specific statements as commands and have them practice with their child. The therapist provides prompting and reinforcement of both the child and the parent.

Calm Follow-Through with Consequences

Another behavioral strategy that we teach parents and use ourselves when addressing any behavioral concern is how to consistently follow through with specific, enforceable consequences. Empty threats do not improve behavior, and helping parents identify consequences they can remember and follow through with is important in the long-term management of children's behavior. HQ Card 3.1 (p. 44) is a summary that can be shared with parents describing these basic behavioral principles. Alternatively, therapists can label small wooden blocks with the principles to serve as visual cues during interventions.

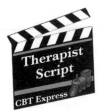

What the Therapist Can Say

"We think of certain behavioral strategies as building blocks. To build new behaviors, we use these blocks [*take out and show labeled wooden blocks or HQ Card 3.1*]— sometimes in different combinations or different orders, but the same basic blocks are used over and over again.

"So, what are those blocks? There are four basic ones we will focus on today: praise, differential attention, effective directions, and calm follow-through with consequences. Depending on the situation, you may start with one block or another. For example, for a behavior like wanting your child to speak more politely to family members, you could start with praise—you praise and comment on each time the child is a little more polite or kind in speaking with others. If you are working on chores, you could start with effective direction and clear expectations first—followed by praise for follow-through. HQ Card 3.1 has some reminders about using these blocks at home."

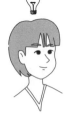

What the Therapist Can Do

Therapists can model the use of these blocks in the room with the family. For example, you can give the child simple commands (*Effective Directions* block) and then reinforce the child's compliance (*Praise* block). Next, therapists should prompt parents to practice these techniques, and they can use the blocks as subtle visual cues to parents about what strategies to try next.

Game Planning for Better Behavior: Defining the Problem and Making a Plan

Ages: Children and parents of children of all ages.

Module: Basic Behavioral Tasks.

Purpose: Clearly define the target behaviors for a behavioral intervention.

Rationale: Parents often have vague strategies for modifying their children's behavior, or they target too many behaviors at once. This *Express* strategy helps keep the family focused on achievable goals.

Materials: HQ Cards 3.2a and 3.2b, Game Planning for Better Behavior, sample and blank cards (pp. 45–46), and a writing utensil.

Expected time needed: 10 minutes.

HQ Cards 3.2a and 3.2b help to quickly guide families to identify and prioritize the behaviors they want to address and to begin to outline specific interventions and how and when to use them. After this is achieved, the next step is to teach caregivers how to respond to compliance and noncompliance. The second section of the HQ Card provides structure and guidance for practicing praise and follow-through with consequences. This technique can be paired with a number of the other Express techniques in this chapter, depending on the parents' knowledge and use of basic behavioral principles. For example, if a parent filling out the HQ Card identifies "decrease saying 'no' when told to do something" as a goal, the provider can work with the parent using Parenting Blocks for Modifying Behavior (see HQ Card 3.1) to promote the use of differential attention, specific praise, and effective directions. Similarly, if a parent identifies "increase my child stopping playing and following directions quickly" as a goal and the child seems to need increased motivation for this behavioral change, the provider can pair this goal with the Inside Out and Outside In intervention (see HQ Cards 3.6a, 3.6b, 3.6c, and 3.6d) to help the family identify ways to boost behavioral changes by adding external motivators.

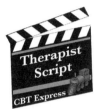

What the Therapist Can Say

"You have described a number of frustrations with your child's behaviors. Knowing where to start can be challenging, and trying to address everything at once will be overwhelming for you and your child. HQ Card 3.2 will help us narrow down the focus to a couple of things to work on first. Once those areas improve, you can use the same approach for other behaviors. Let's take a look at this together and see if we can identify a few behaviors with which you would like to start. How does that sound?"

The therapist acknowledges the parent's frustrations and desire to change the child's behavior and quickly transitions to the *Express* intervention. You can show you have heard the scope of the parent's concerns by acknowledging there are more behaviors than can be covered all at once, while pointing out that the strategies that will be addressed can be generalized to other behaviors as well. Finally, the therapist works collaboratively with the parent to identify which behaviors the family wants to start with rather than dictating those for the family.

Tell, Show, Rehearse, Review, and Repeat

Ages: Parents of children of all ages.

Module: Psychoeducation; Basic Behavioral Tasks.

Purpose: Teach, model, rehearse, and reinforce parental use of behavioral interventions.

Rationale: Simply telling parents about behavioral strategies will lead to limited utilization of the techniques. By having the strategies modeled and practicing the techniques during the visit, families are more likely to gain understanding of and therefore use the strategies outside of session.

Materials: None.

Expected time needed: 15 minutes.

When working with families to identify behavioral goals, you will likely discover you need to provide brief but specific training on effective behavioral interventions. Examples include training caregivers on the use of differential attention, specific praise, effective directions, and follow-through with consequences.

Overall, there are five simple steps to training caregivers to shape children's behavior:

1. Tell.
2. Show.
3. Rehearse.
4. Review.
5. Repeat.

Step 1 is psychoeducation, the Tell step. Parents may need very specific education on basic behavioral principles. We caution providers to keep these descriptions short and relevant during *Express* interventions. Start with one or two principles and use examples from the family's own history or from what you have observed in the room with the family. For example, if describing the benefits of praise for increasing a child's positive behaviors, you can talk with parents about how telling the child how nicely she is sitting still can lead to more sitting still.

Step 2 is Show, which means you need to model and practice the strategies with the family. For example, parents often say, "I tell him to do something, and he just won't do it," but then if you observe the parent interacting with the child, the parent is often using vague instructions or questions rather than specific and direct commands: "John can you pick up your stuff? John, do you hear me? Can you pick up your stuff like I asked? John? JOHN?"

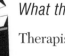

What the Therapist Can Say

Therapists can introduce the Show step by saying the following:

"Now that we have talked about how praise can improve your child's behaviors and help increase the frequency with which he listens to you, let me show you what I mean. I see that he has been sitting quietly looking at that book while we were talking. I would say to him, "Thank you for sitting so quietly and patiently waiting while I talk with your parents." Did you notice how he grinned when I just said that? In a few minutes you could praise him again to further reinforce these behaviors, and therefore increase the chances he will continue to sit quietly."

Once you have described the strategy to parents (Tell) and modeled it (Show), it is time for practice (the Rehearse step). The interactions between parent and child represent long-standing habits. Changing these patterns will not be a simple feat and will not occur after just one practice. It will be important for you to continue to model the strategies throughout interactions, and to continue to explicitly point out what you are doing and how the child is responding.

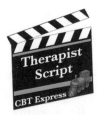

What the Therapist Can Say

"You saw how I praised John for sitting quietly, now I want you to practice pointing out the things he is doing well. What behaviors do you notice him doing now that you can point out to him and praise him for?"

Sometimes parents will struggle with finding specific behaviors to praise, and you may have to circle back to Step 1 and provide more teaching, or offer visual cues (e.g., a note card with a few target behaviors to praise or a few examples of praise statements). After completing Steps 1, 2, and 3, you will be ready for Step 4, Review. You should review or summarize what was done and the impact it has had on the child.

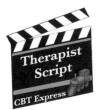

What the Therapist Can Say

"What did you notice during that interaction with John? How did he respond when you pointed out he was sitting so quietly? When do you think you can use this strategy at home?"

Finally, you arrive at Step 5, which is to Repeat this process with other behavioral strategies as needed to help build parental understanding and use of behavior modification techniques. Such strategies might include giving specific directions, ignoring/differential attention, and shaping of behaviors.

The Homework Balance (After-School Schedule)

Ages: School age.

Module: Basic Behavioral Tasks.

Purpose: Provide clear expectations and strategies for time management around homework completion.

Rationale: Many children lack independent skills in time management. With clear expectations and a realistic schedule, the entire family will be less frustrated with homework time.

Materials: HQ Card 3.3, The Homework Balance (After-School Schedule) (p. 47), and a writing utensil.

Expected time needed: 5–10 minutes.

A frequent battle in any family is homework completion. Parents often want their children/teens to be more independent, motivated, and efficient in doing their homework. When children or teens don't finish their homework, parents get angry and punish the child, which can lead to arguments and frustration for the entire family.

When families express concern with this behavioral pattern, defining realistic expectations and helping family members view each other's perspectives can be helpful in balancing the parent's and child's priorities. Some parents overestimate their children's skills, self-control, and time management. They expect the child to manage her own after-school schedule and homework load. At the time when they are supposed to do homework (evening hours), children can be tired and hungry after a full day of school, after-school activities, day care, or after-school jobs. Parents are also likely exhausted from their day. Families who have already established a pattern of battling over homework may not realize how the small things they say and do can be perpetuating this pattern.

It is no surprise that having a schedule can help improve success in completing desired tasks after school. That being said, many families do not have explicit expectations for the schedule. Therefore, parents may have their own thoughts about what the schedule should be and teens or children have their own thoughts too, but they have not discussed the schedule in detail with each other. Take the following discussion with Carolina and her mother, for example. Mom has clear ideas about what Carolina should do after school. The therapist must work with Mom on flexibility and then on follow-through so that in the end Carolina is more likely to follow the agreed-upon homework schedule.

THERAPIST: You indicated on the visit paperwork that homework is a concern. What is most difficult about homework?

MOM: She never wants to do it. She just comes home, locks her door, and gets right on her phone.

CAROLINA: I just want to relax for a little bit after school—but she's all over me, banging on the door, asking me when I am coming out and getting started on homework.

THERAPIST: It sounds like you each have different ideas about what should happen after school and not agreeing with the other's ideas leaves you arguing. If you both had the same expectations for after school, and you both agreed to following the rules we set up, you might avoid the arguing. Can we give it a try?

MOM: What do you mean? She has to do her homework. That is not negotiable.

THERAPIST: True, but perhaps if we set up rules about when she does the work and with what reminders or rules around it, then we can untangle this nightly argument. Are you both willing to spend the next 5 minutes trying to set a couple of basic rules?

CAROLINA AND MOM: Sure. I guess.

THERAPIST: OK, so we have established that Carolina wants to relax after school and Mom wants her to do her homework. Carolina, what do you think is a reasonable amount of time to relax after school before starting homework?

CAROLINA: An hour. I just really need to unwind.

MOM: That won't work because on Tuesdays you have dance right after dinner, so if you don't start your homework sooner, you won't finish in time.

THERAPIST: OK, so what about on Mondays and Wednesdays? Anywhere Carolina has to be those nights?

MOM: Not right now.

THERAPIST: OK, so on Mondays and Wednesday if Carolina gets home at 4:15 and relaxes for an hour, then starts homework, would that be acceptable to you, Mom?

MOM: Sure, if she actually did it—but that is doubtful.

THERAPIST: We will worry about that in a minute, right now we just want to set up what is fair. Carolina, does an hour of relaxation time on Mondays and Wednesdays seem fair to you?

CAROLINA: Sure, if she actually left me alone and didn't keep pounding on my door asking me what I am doing.

The therapist starts by getting the family engaged in a discussion about a realistic time frame. Carolina has the flexibility to have an hour of "free time" 2 days a week. Once she has a response to her desire for downtime, Carolina feels heard and the family is on the path toward a schedule on which they can all agree. Next, the therapist needs to work with the family on outlining expectations for the other days. Phase 2 will involve implementing this plan and defining the consequences for following or not following the agreed-upon schedule. Parenting Blocks can be used to augment this intervention and help nudge parents to use behavioral interventions during the setting of the schedule. HQ Card 3.3 can assist families in outlining the details of the schedule and then tracking compliance with each step, both to monitor for progress as well as to provide opportunities for reinforcing successful completion of steps.

Homework Battle Defuser

Ages: School age.

Modules: Psychoeducation; Basic Behavioral Tasks.

Purpose: Identify motivators for task completion.

Rationale: Many children lack internal motivation to complete homework. Identification and effective use of external motivators can increase homework completion and reduce parent–child conflict.

Materials: HQ Card 3.4, Homework Battle Defuser (p. 48).

Expected time needed: 5–10 minutes.

For many children, homework is overwhelming and they struggle with motivation to get the work done. If school is challenging, they don't understand assignments, or they see little value in the assignments, they may resist the homework even more. Further, children with learning disabilities or executive function difficulties may struggle more than the typical child or teen with getting work done. Those factors coupled with other enticing distractions, such as electronics, friends, and hobbies, can result in a recipe for parent–child conflict and nightly battles over homework. Therapists may need to work with children and their families to break down the homework struggles and figure out which ingredients are key in their individual family's homework battle. Specifically, what makes the homework difficult? Is it lack of skill or poor understanding of the tasks? Is it low motivation on the part of the child? Does chaos or noise in the home make concentration difficult? Is the child hungry or tired, leading to fewer emotional and cognitive reserves to complete tasks independently?

Once some of the key elements to the battle have been identified through this *Express* technique, the therapist can work with the family to defuse the battles with more collaborative problem solving, productive discussions, and family rules about homework time. External motivators and basic agreement on realistic expectations can be important and effective ingredients to add in as well. HQ Card 3.4 can be used with families to outline specifics and begin modifying the plan.

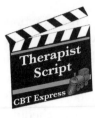

What the Therapist Can Say

"It is tough getting motivated to do something that is challenging or not fun. From what you described, there are several battles around homework avoidance that we want to defuse. She is often tired and grumpy during homework time, and chooses electronics over studying. She doesn't naturally have the drive or desire to do the homework at that time. HQ Card 3.4 will help us identify what can motivate her to do the work by providing clear expectations and rewards. These expectations and rewards are the new key pieces that will reduce the homework battles!"

What the Therapist Can Do

Therapists can use HQ Card 3.4 to help families outline the current "battles" and identify replacements to improve homework time and defuse the homework battles into more manageable tasks.

Simon Says "Chore Time"

Ages: 3 years through teens.

Module: Basic behavioral tasks.

Purpose: Increase compliance with daily chores.

Rationale: Parental complaints that children are noncompliant with chores typically reflect a larger compliance issue. If parents increase their use of effective commands and praise, children will become more compliant with simple tasks, and eventually with more complex chores.

Materials: Items around the office or home, HQ Card 3.5, Simon Says "Chore Time" (p. 49).

Expected time needed: 5 minutes.

Whether it is an office or a clinic exam room, the environment where you see families offers countless temptations for the curious child. When parents are already challenged by their children's behavior, there's nothing like trying to stop them from spinning a wheeled chair or stool or ripping up the paper on an exam table to elevate their frustration. For a therapist, these moments provide an ideal in vivo opportunity for an *Express* intervention to show how to apply behavior modification strategies. These situations allow for a chance at meaningful practice of newly taught techniques. The therapist can also observe how the child responds, and then modify the approach if needed.

Sometimes providers shy away from coaching parents to practice behavioral techniques in real time. It can feel awkward, and it is definitely easier to talk about what to do than to actually do it. However, the benefits of the real-life practice cannot be understated. When a parent observes the provider giving an effective command and then observes the child following the command, this not only models how adults can word things and respond to both compliance and noncompliance, it also shows parents that their child is capable of complying with the help of certain interventions. If the child melts down or refuses, it can feel validating for parents to "show" the therapist what they have been talking about, but it is also a prime opportunity to acknowledge the parents' frustration and for the therapist to demonstrate for the parents how to respond to such behaviors in a calm and effective manner. The dialogue below offers an example.

> THERAPIST: Last week you mentioned that CJ "never listens" to the things you tell him to do, especially helping with chores around the house. Today I thought we could spend a few minutes trying to change how the directions are given and see if that makes a difference in CJ's behavior.
>
> MOM: I guess, but he doesn't listen to anyone.
>
> THERAPIST: When a child doesn't follow directions, it can start to seem like we have no way of changing that pattern. Let's see if we can get some change today. CJ, please hand me that box of tissues next to you.
>
> CJ: (*Looks up from his video game and pushes the tissue box across the counter to the therapist.*)
>
> THERAPIST: Hey, thanks for following directions so quickly!
>
> MOM: I'm surprised he did that so quickly, but that is also not the same as a chore.
>
> CJ: (*Briefly looks up from his game and rolls his eyes.*)
>
> THERAPIST: True, but if we get CJ to follow simple directions more often, it might make the more complex ones like chores easier too. It is kind of like when he was learning to talk—you didn't expect full sentences right away. Early on, if he said a word or anything that sounded like a word, what did you do?
>
> MOM: We would cheer and repeat the word. Clap with him. We made a big deal of it.
>
> THERAPIST: Right. And once he was saying lots of words did you keep cheering every time?
>
> MOM: No, we made more of a big deal if he asked a question or said something new.
>
> THERAPIST: We want to work on starting with the simple directions, kind of like starting with simple words, and then work up to chores and complex direction like you worked up to sentences when CJ was learning to talk.
>
> MOM: I guess that makes sense.
>
> THERAPIST: If we give simple directions and then praise CJ and reward him for following the directions, we can eventually work up to the more complex ones. (*Takes a tissue from the box and passes the box back to CJ*). Thanks, CJ. Put the tissues back where they were.
>
> CJ: (*Ignores direction and keeps playing his game.*)
>
> THERAPIST: CJ, you need to either put the tissues back where they were or stop playing your game. Your choice.
>
> CJ: (*Rolls his eyes, and then without looking up slides the tissues back in place.*)
>
> THERAPIST: Good choice and following directions.

Some children will begrudgingly go along with these demonstrations, and others will be eager for the positive attention and react playfully. For younger and more engaged children, a "Simon Says" type of game can be used. Giving the child several directions in a row that are fun but specific helps the child practice doing something he or she is told to do, and for many children who have been bored waiting in an exam room or stuck in a hospital room, it is a welcome distraction. Consider 4-year-old Carli, who was seen in a primary care clinic during a well-child check. The clinic was running behind, and she had been in the room for quite a while. When the therapist came in, Carli was fidgety and kept trying to turn on the water at the sink. Her mother was frustrated that she had to keep telling her "over and over again" to "get away from the sink." Carli's mom was eager to share her frustrations.

MOM: Carli won't listen. She makes a mess everywhere and when I tell her to clean up she just walks away or gets something else out. As you can see, she won't even listen in here. She won't leave that sink alone . . . just wants to be in the water.

THERAPIST: It's tough in these rooms—the water and the spinning stools are so tempting. And it sounds frustrating to have to tell her the same things over and over again.

MOM: Yes, it sure is! She just won't stop.

THERAPIST: Would it be OK if we tried a few things in here to see if we can get Carli to listen and do what you say more?

MOM: Sure.

THERAPIST: OK. We are going to focus on two things. First, telling Carli short things to do and second praising her for doing them quickly. Remember the game Simon Says? We will kind of take that approach of telling her simple fun things quickly. Let's see how she responds. (*Turns her attention to Carli.*) Carli, clap your hands. (*Therapist demonstrates clapping. Carli begins clapping and smiling.*) Good listening, Carli! Now jump. (*Therapist demonstrates a small hop. Carli begins jumping.*) You are following directions so nicely! (*Gives Carli a high-5 and Carli smiles.*) Carli, touch your toes. Excellent listening. Stand up straight. Good work standing straight. Now sit in that chair. Wow, you follow directions so well (*high-5*). Mom, now your turn.

MOM: Carli, clap your hands. (*Carli just looks at her mom.*) Clap, Carli, clap your hands. (*Mom begins clapping and Carli claps once. Mom is quiet.*)

THERAPIST: (*Whispers to Mom.*) Tell her "Good job following directions."

MOM: Good job following directions, Carli. Now stand up. (*Carli slowly stands. Therapist nods at Mom to indicate it is time to praise.*) Good job listening, Carli. Now, Carli, hop up and down. (*Carli hops.*) Good job hopping, Carli.

THERAPIST: Excellent, you are giving very specific and short directions, praising Carli each time and she is doing it! After a while, she may get bored hearing the same thing over and over ("Good job, good job"), so we can use HQ Card 3.5 to think of a few different ways to praise her to keep her interested. (*Works with Mom to complete the worksheet.*) So what do you think about practicing this at home?

MOM: She seems to like it, but what about when I need to her clean up her toys or pick up her clothes? Then it isn't a game anymore.

THERAPIST: I wonder how she would respond if it seemed more like a game or if we tried telling her to do those things in the same way we just did the clapping and hopping. Let's take this paper towel and give it a try, OK?

MOM: OK.

THERAPIST: (*Rips up a paper towel and scatters the pieces on the floor.*) OK, let's try this and see how it goes. (*Mom nods.*) Carli, touch your nose—That's right! I like how quickly you listened to directions. Now do a jumping jack. Very nice following directions (*high-5*). Carli, pick up those pieces of paper towel and throw them in that trash can (*pointing*). (*Carli slowly bends down by one of the pieces and is reaching for it.*) Carli, you are listening so quickly—wow, good job cleaning up the towels . . . you are following directions well. . . . (*as Carli picks them up*).

MOM: Hmmmm, I am surprised she did that.

THERAPIST: What did you notice about Carli when I told her to pick up the paper towels?

MOM: She was moving kind of slowly and just looked at you at first but then she did it.

THERAPIST: Yeah, I noticed that too—she seemed to be thinking about it before she did it! You may have also noticed I praised her as soon as she started picking them up, rather than waiting until she was done.

MOM: Yeah, I don't think I would have thought to do that. I would have waited, but it seems to have helped her keep going.

THERAPIST: Exactly. That little bit of praise once she started cleaning up was like the fuel that took her to the next step, and so on. Eventually you won't need to praise her every step of the way, but for now that is what will help motivate her and remind her at the same time about what she is supposed to be doing.

MOM: Let me see if she will do it with me. (*Mom practices with Carli.*)

This dialogue illustrates several key parts of intervening to improve Carli's behavior. The exchange includes direct instruction for mom on the use of behavioral interventions. It also includes the therapist modeling the techniques, and then coaching and reinforcing mom's efforts while she practices with Carlie. These interactions also help build a positive relationship between Carli and her mother, and resulted in both parent and child attending more to the positive behaviors and interactions. The exercise creates more positive exchanges that may not have been occurring otherwise. HQ Card 3.5 offers some examples of directions and praise parents can refer to while learning and practicing the Simon Says *Express* technique. Therapists may also want to pair the Parenting Blocks for Modifying Behavior with this technique to reinforce the strategies in the future.

Inside Out and Outside In

Ages: All ages.

Module: Basic Behavioral Tasks.

Purpose: Increase motivation for desired tasks using external motivators.

Rationale: Parents often want children to want to do chores and other less desirable tasks. This Express intervention helps parents understand the difference between internal and external motivation, as well as use external motivators to increase desired behaviors.

Materials: HQ Cards 3.6a, 3.6b, 3.6c, and 3.6d, Inside Out and Outside In, samples and blank cards (pp. 50–53), and a writing utensil.

Expected time needed: 10–15 minutes.

> "She's just lazy."
>
> "He never wants to do anything besides what he wants to do."
>
> "All he does is watch TV and play video games."
>
> "I can't get her to do anything. Everything is in slow motion."

These are some of the common comments we hear from parents of children who seem to have low motivation and/or low energy. These children often lack internal motivation to complete less desirable tasks, such as schoolwork, chores, and activities of daily living. Helping parents get past the frustration, and focus on strategies to increase action by children is the challenge to therapists.

THERAPIST: You mentioned that Kyra has a hard time getting moving, and you find yourself having to "nag" her every day to do the basic tasks you expect of her.

MOM: That's right. She won't do the simplest things, like pick her dirty clothes up off the bathroom floor, without being told to do so. I even put a basket in the bathroom, and she leaves her clothes right next to the basket! It is ridiculous.

THERAPIST: Sounds challenging.

MOM: It is. I don't understand why she doesn't want to help out more. She should notice the dishwasher needs unloading and just unload it, but she never does unless I tell her to several times.

THERAPIST: One thing that is important to know when trying to get kids to do things is whether they are motivated by things "inside" or "outside." For some tasks, Kyra may not need to be reminded to do them—she just does them because she wants to or it is important to her. We call this "intrinsic" motivation: she is motivated internally or by something inside her.

MOM: Sure, like using her phone or doing her hair.

THERAPIST: Socializing and self-care tasks may be motivating to Kyra by themselves because she finds the time with friends enjoyable, so that is reinforcing and motivating. It is like something inside her makes her want to do the activity. But there are other things she doesn't find reinforcing or "fun," so she has more trouble getting started or completing those things.

MOM: Yeah, like pretty much everything else.

THERAPIST: For some tasks that are less internally motivating, we may need to create a motivation for Kyra outside of her own feelings or drive to do the task.

MOM: So, give her something for doing what she is supposed to do?

THERAPIST: We can use what is important to Kyra as a reward or motivator for her doing what she needs to do but is less motivated to do. For example, you mentioned she is motivated to use her phone but she is often slow with getting things ready to get out the door for school in the morning. So, she has the inner drive or what we call internal motivation to use her phone, but not to get ready quickly for school. If we set it up so she has to complete certain steps for getting ready before she gets her phone in the mornings, we are taking something outside of her (the use of the phone) to create a motivation to do something she has no "inside" motivation to do.

MOM: You want me to bribe her to get ready for school?

THERAPIST: We want to show her that it is beneficial to her to get ready for school [something she is not motivated to do] because she will get to use her phone if she does [something she is highly motivated to do]. It is basically giving her a choice by telling her what will happen—if you do X you get Y.

MOM: OK, she might do that because she likes to listen to music on her phone on the bus in the mornings, and she will probably want to be texting with her friends too.

THERAPIST: Let's outline what other things might be motivating on the outside that we can put in place to get Kyra to do the things she isn't motivated to do on the inside [see HQ Card 3.6a]. It is like turning things outside in and inside out.

Next, we want to bring in the motivators so that the connection between difficult tasks and reinforcers is developed and the reinforcing things (use of phone) will help with the completion of less desirable activities (homework) (see HQ Card 3.6b).

Conclusion

When working with families on noncompliance and motivating children and teens, the frustration caregivers experience is often evident in both what the caregivers express to the provider as well as how they respond to and interact with the child. Helping caregivers focus on the behavioral changes and remain unemotional in their reaction to the child's frustrating behavior is no small feat. As a provider, you must be supportive and understanding of the frustrations, while teaching caregivers effective alternatives. Some of the *Express* strategies introduced earlier in this chapter will be helpful, such as the use of effective directions and praise. When caregivers have specific steps to follow, they are more likely to feel in control and effective in their parenting skills. If we can give caregivers the key building blocks to success, they are more likely to use those in new situations after treatment has discontinued.

Building Blocks

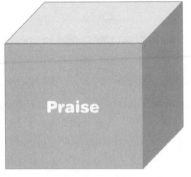

Praise: Tell your child EXACTLY what he or she is doing that you like and want to see more of.

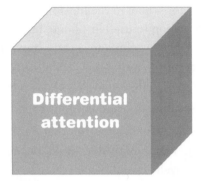

Differential attention: Whatever behavior you give attention to will occur more often!

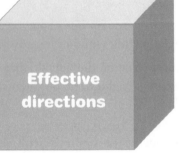

Effective directions: Give short, specific statements (not questions!). If someone can answer yes or no, it is a question.

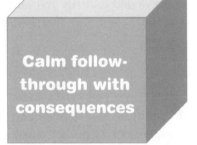

Calm follow-through with consequences: Give specific, short-term consequences for misbehavior. Avoid threats and multiple warnings.

Game Planning for Better Behavior: Sample

Where to start?: *Identifying your top three targets*

Put a ✓ next to the one to three behaviors that you want to change first:

☑ Says "No" when told to do something

☐ Ignores and keeps playing when told to do something

☑ Stops playing and follows directions within a few minutes of being told

☐ Yells at parents/caregivers

☐ Throws things

☐ Hugs or gives loving touches to family members

☐ Rolls eyes

☑ Other (specify): <u>walks away when I am talking to him</u>

Making the right moves:

To increase behaviors you want to see more often, praise or reward your child every time he or she engages in that behavior.

To decrease behaviors you want to see less often, praise or reward the opposite behavior.

1. To   increase   / (decrease) <u>saying "no" when told to do something</u>

   I will <u>say "thank you for following directions" each time he does what I said</u>.

   When my child does <u>say "no"</u>

   I will <u>give him a choice to do as I said or go to his room for a time-out</u>.

2. To (increase) /   decrease   <u>my child stopping playing and following directions quickly</u>

   I will <u>praise him each time he does so ("I like when you follow directions quickly.")</u>.

   When my child does <u>not stop playing</u>

   I will <u>let him know the consequences (you need to take a break from playing and set the table now or you will be done playing video games for the rest of the evening)</u>.

3. To   increase   / (decrease) <u>my child walking away when I am talking to him</u>

   I will <u>give short and specific directions and praise him for listening respectfully</u>.

   When my child does <u>walk away</u>

   I will <u>tell him to stop and listen or he will be given extra chores</u>.

Game Planning for Better Behavior

Where to start?: *Identifying your top three targets*

Put a ✓ next to the one to three behaviors that you want to change first:

☐ Says "No" when told to do something

☐ Ignores and keeps playing when told to do something

☐ Stops playing and follows directions within a few minutes of being told

☐ Yells at parents/caregivers

☐ Throws things

☐ Hugs or gives loving touches to family members

☐ Rolls eyes

☐ Other (specify): _____

Making the right moves:

To increase behaviors you want to see more often, praise or reward your child every time he or she engages in that behavior.

To decrease behaviors you want to see less often, praise or reward the opposite behavior.

1. To increase / decrease _____

   I will _____.

   When my child does _____

   I will _____.

2. To increase / decrease _____

   I will _____.

   When my child does _____

   I will _____.

3. To increase / decrease _____

   I will _____.

   When my child does _____

   I will _____.

The Homework Balance (After-School Schedule)

Example

4:00–4:15	Get home, get settled, have a snack	
4:15–4:30	Relax, text friends	
4:30–4:45	Relax, text friends	
4:45–5:00	Relax, text friends	
5:00–5:15	Relax, text friends	
5:15–5:30	Help Mom get table set	
5:30–5:45	Homework	
5:45–6:00	Homework	
6:00–6:15	Homework	
6:15–6:30	Dinner	
6:30–6:45	Dinner, help clean up	
6:45–7:00	Homework	
7:00–7:15	Homework	
7:15–7:30	Homework	
7:30–7:45	Break	
7:45–8:00	Homework	

Fill in your schedule below.

4:00–4:15		
4:15–4:30		
4:30–4:45		
4:45–5:00		
5:00–5:15		
5:15–5:30		
5:30–5:45		
5:45–6:00		
6:00–6:15		
6:15–6:30		
6:30–6:45		
6:45–7:00		
7:00–7:15		
7:15–7:30		
7:30–7:45		
7:45–8:00		

Homework Battle Defuser

Our current homework battles include:

_____ Phone/text distractions during homework time

_____ Feeling tired after school

_____ Feeling hungry after school

_____ Not understanding the work

_____ Have a set after-school schedule

_____ Cellphone turned off during homework time

_____ Reward for completion of homework

_____ Other: _____

We will defuse the battles with the following:

_____ Have a set after-school schedule

_____ Cellphone turned off during homework time

_____ Reward for completion of homework

_____ Snack after school

_____ Tutoring by teacher during study hall

_____ Doing homework in different location: _____

_____ Other: _____

Simon Says "Chore Time"

See the examples below and then add some ideas of your own.

Direction	Ideas for Praise
Clap your hands.	Good job listening.
Jump.	Nice work following directions.
Sit down.	I like how you listened so quickly.
Stand up.	You did that so fast!
Touch your toes.	You are following directions nicely.
Put this (item) on the table.	Wow, you are following directions well.
Throw this in the trash.	Excellent work cleaning up.
Hand me (item).	Great job (insert direction).

Inside Out and Outside In: Sample

Put the things in the big circle that are motivating and easy to do. Put things in the smaller circle that are not motivating or are harder to do.

Homework

Unloading the dishwasher

Picking up dirty clothes

Texting friends

Walking the dog/playing with the dog

Helping with cooking

Inside Out and Outside In: Sample Connecting the Circles

By connecting the big and small circles, we can help children complete less motivating tasks using highly motivating rewards.

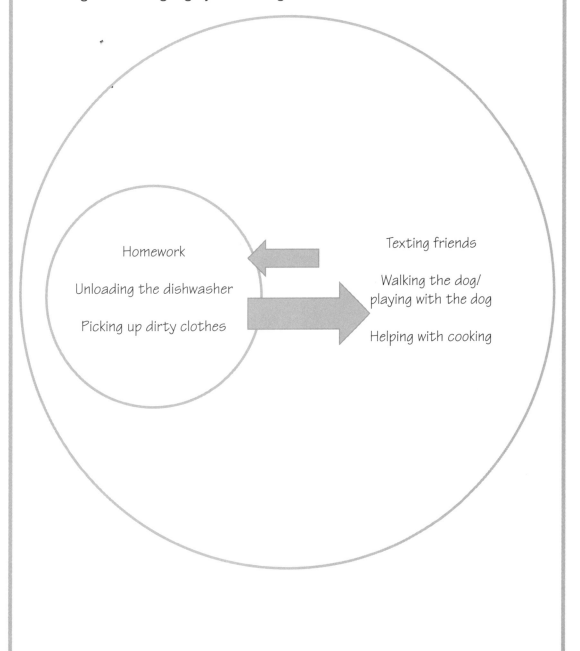

Homework

Unloading the dishwasher

Picking up dirty clothes

Texting friends

Walking the dog/ playing with the dog

Helping with cooking

Inside Out and Outside In

Put the things in the big circle that are motivating and easy to do. Put things in the smaller circle that are not motivating or are harder to do.

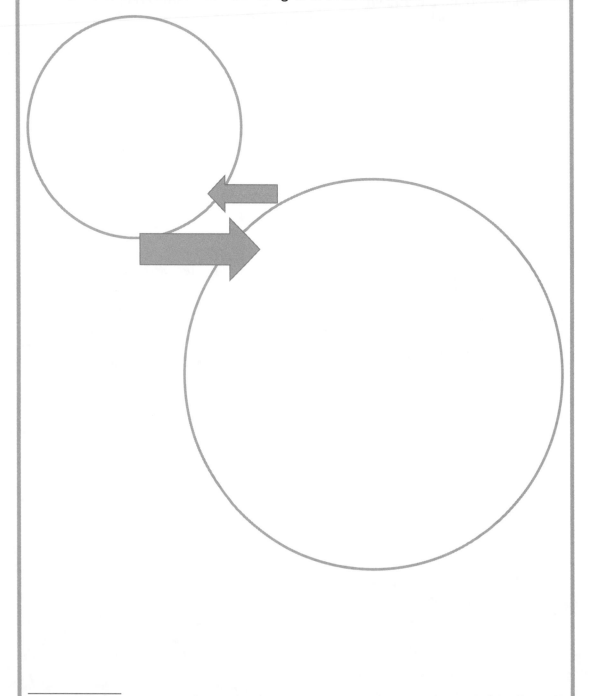

Inside Out and Outside In: Connecting the Circles

By connecting the big and small circles, we can help children complete less motivating tasks using highly motivating rewards.

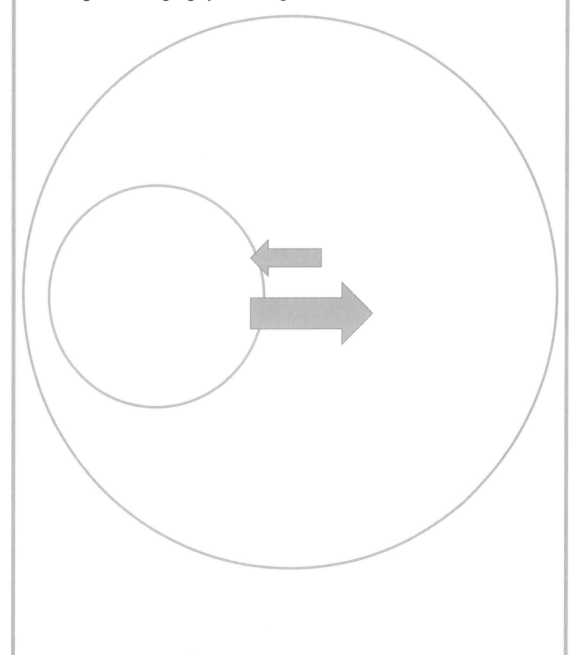

Anger

"Anytime she doesn't get her way it is like a light switch. She flips from fine to explosion."

"He's so easily offended. It is like he thinks everyone is out to get him and he gets mad at them so easily."

"He has anger issues."

"She lashes out at others."

Like all feelings, anger is a typical experience for children. It is when the degree and frequency of the anger, often coupled with verbal or physical aggression, causes problems that it is brought to the attention of physicians, school counselors, psychologists, or other providers. These externalizing behaviors lead to social problems, get kids in trouble at school or daycare, and lead to family conflict. Typically, anger does not occur in isolation. Impulse control issues can lead to more aggression when a child is angered, and mood disturbance can cause cognitive distortions that reinforce negative thoughts and anger patterns. Disruptive home life can trigger more anger, and caregiver modeling can impact the pattern as well.

Brief Statement Regarding Evidence-Based Treatments

Angry behaviors like yelling, fighting, and arguing get kids in trouble and irritate parents. Youth often react with anger when they think they are being treated unfairly or they misunderstand a situation. CBT is shown to effectively address each of these skills deficits and behavioral excesses. Behavioral interventions teach youth ways to calm themselves down and react differently to their anger (Landenberger & Lipsey, 2005). Cognitive strategies generate improvements in problem-solving skills, and kids learn to reappraise situations to limit hostile responses (Lochman & Wells, 2002). For young patients who struggle with peer conflict, learning social skills like compromise, negotiation, and communication is an important element of treatment (Hammond & Yung, 1991; Lochman et al., 2011). Relational aggression is increasingly important to address given the wide variety of social media platforms and the substantial amount of interaction that occurs via mobile devices (Görzig & Frumkin, 2013). Emotionally evocative in-session practices (exposures) are critical as they facilitate skill generalization and capitalize on state-dependent learning (Goldstein et al., 2013; Lochman & Wells, 2002). It is also important to incorporate caregivers into therapy so that they can support skill application and coach youth in everyday settings (McCart & Sheidow, 2016; Smith, Lochman, & Daunic, 2005).

CBT is an effective treatment for angry behaviors for youth of all ages. Youth who learn and apply CBT skills show improved social functioning, better academic performance, decreased problem behaviors, less frequent peer rejection, and enhanced understanding of social situations (Goldstein et al., 2013; Lochman et al., 2011; Lochman & Wells, 2002, 2003). Youth also show better comprehension of their emotions and improved perspective taking (Lochman et al., 2011). Gains are shown to be maintained up to 3 years in some studies (McCart & Sheidow, 2016). Long-term benefits of CBT for angry behaviors included reduced risk for substance abuse, legal problems, and truancy (Lochman & Wells, 2002). Although the majority of research is completed with males, several studies show that the same strategies apply to therapy with females (Goldstein et al., 2013). CBT tools work equally well for young children as with adolescents and are applicable across ethnicities and socioeconomic statuses (Hammond & Yung, 1991; Martinez & Eddy, 2005; McCart & Sheidow, 2016). Because angry behaviors can occur with youth facing any number of problems, *CBT Express* strategies give providers a way to directly intervene for troubling behavior patterns and introduce new skills in a variety of settings.

Presenting Concerns and Symptoms

Parents use the term *anger* when describing a number of behaviors they are observing in their children. Most commonly, parents describe observing yelling, back talking, and facial expressions indicating frustration and anger on the part of their child. Some children also engage in physical aggression, lashing out at others or destroying property. The interventions in this chapter are designed to address mild to moderate behaviors associated with anger, such as yelling, shouting, back talking, and mild aggression.

Interventions

A youth's anger outbursts are generally described by parents as typically being preceded by an observable behavior. Therefore, many interventions we recommend are implemented at the point of this trigger, or prior to the "angry behaviors." In addition, how the parent responds to a display of anger by a child can reinforce the child's behaviors, so parents need to be cognizant of the behaviors to which they are attending.

After reading Chapter 2, readers should be familiar with the ABC's of children's problems. For children and their caregivers to address behaviors indicative of anger or anger outbursts, we present interventions to target the anger triggers and reactions to the triggers.

Double Dribble

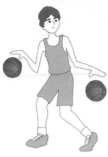

Ages: 6 years and older.

Module: Psychoeducation.

Purpose: Increase identification of behaviors and consequences of behaviors, and increase motivation to engage in other intervention strategies.

Rationale: Children do not often stop and think about the consequences of their actions. Therefore, when they receive a consequence for a behavior, they may become even angrier (angry about the initial anger trigger as well as the consequence for their own behaviors).

Materials: HQ Card 4.1, Double Dribble (p. 72), and writing utensil.

Expected time needed: 2 minutes.

Often children lack an understanding of how the consequences of their own behaviors are contributing to their frustrations. Patterns that are so clear to caregivers go unrecognized by the children. Double Dribble brings to light the repetitive patterns angry children may find themselves in—engaging in the same behaviors over and over and getting frustrated by the consequences. This *Express* strategy is designed to shed some light on those patterns, thus motivating the youth to engage in other interventions presented in this chapter.

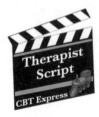

What the Therapist Can Say

"Do you know how to dribble a basketball? What do you have to do if you are dribbling and then stop dribbling? That's right, you have to do something different than dribbling. You can pass the ball to a teammate, or try to shoot a basket. Dribbling again is against the rules and will result in a 'double dribble' call, and the other team will get the ball.

Your anger reactions are kind of like a double dribble. You can keep doing the same thing you have always done, but it doesn't end well. Or you can try something different, like passing the ball or taking a shot at the basket, and take a chance at a better outcome. We want to try and do something different with your anger. Instead of dribbling again, we want to try another strategy."

Depending on how much time the provider has with the child that day, he or she can then move into one of the following interventions or can make plans to do so at the next visit. This strategy provides a quick introduction to the idea that things can be different and helps the child start to see that he may have some control or influence over what happens if he chooses to change his behaviors. This 2-minute intervention can be enhanced with demonstrations of dribbling a small ball or a video of double dribbling during a basketball game.

Assertive Anger

Ages: 8 years and older.

Module: Psychoeducation.

Purpose: Learn how to assertively express angry feelings.

Rationale: Many youth lack the basic skill of communicating their emotions clearly and assertively. Without this skill, youth will only be able to stay calm for so long—either resorting to aggressive anger expressions or getting into a suppression/explosion cycle. Explicit training on assertive communication fills this skill vacuum.

Materials: HQ Card 4.2, Assertive Anger (p. 73), and a writing utensil.

Expected time needed: 15 minutes.

Even if children are able to use self-regulation strategies to remain calm in the face of anger triggers, unless they learn how to appropriately express their frustration, they will return to previous angry reactions. Thus, effective coaching includes both ideas for how to stay calm as well as assertive communication of their anger. Not all anger needs to be expressed, so we recommend that children begin to practice this skill with adults only (i.e., caregivers, teachers). Once youth master the ability to assertively communicate their anger, they may begin to identify when it is a good idea to express anger toward peers.

Consider the example of Terry, who was referred for treatment due to anger outbursts. The counselor is working with Terry on how to demonstrate the skill of effectively communicating. In the following dialogue, Terry and his counselor use Assertive Anger to identify different ways Terry can express his anger without hurting others or getting himself into trouble.

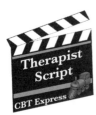

What the Therapist Can Say

COUNSELOR: You are working hard to effectively communicate when you feel angry. This next worksheet is going to teach you how to tell Mom what made you so mad when she told you "no" about going to the game Thursday night with your friend.

TERRY: She already knows what makes me mad.

COUNSELOR: Are you sure? Because to be honest, I'm not sure I know what you are angry about. Other than missing out on the game, of course. I mean, you could be mad that you don't get to stay up late, or that your friend will get to hang out with someone else, or because he is going to call you a baby because you can't go out on a school night.

TERRY: All right, all right I get it.

COUNSELOR: OK, so if you look at this paper, you can see there are already ideas of how to start. We are just going to go through and fill in the different pieces with your specific thoughts.

The tricky part about learning to express yourself assertively is that it does not guarantee you will get what you want. It is important to emphasize to youth when training this skill that this is *not* about getting what they want, it's about making sure the other person understands how they feel. When people understand us, we end up feeling less frustrated and we get into trouble less often.

Roll the Dice

Ages: 5 years and older.

Module: Psychoeducation.

Purpose: Improve child's awareness of and appropriate expression of various emotions.

Rationale: Children often respond with anger when they are uncomfortable with or do not know how to express other emotions. Roll the Dice provides a fun way to teach and practice feeling identification and expression with children and families.

Materials: Dice and HQ Card 4.3, Roll the Dice (p. 74). *Alternative: Create your own feeling dice as described below.*

Expected time needed: 10 minutes.

Some children who struggle with anger are uncomfortable or lack the skills to appropriately identify and express other feelings. When they become frustrated with a task, feel left out by peers, or are nervous in a new setting, they are not able to articulate their feelings. Anger can be more prevalent, therefore, in those situations. Roll the Dice helps build skills in feeling identification and expression, as well as promoting communication of feelings between the child and caregivers. Strengthening these skills can normalize expression of feelings and increase the level of communication between the child and family members about various feelings. Parents' modeling of appropriate feeling expression can also be powerful.

Roll the Dice requires some prep work by the provider in order to be ready when a particular child may need this technique. Taking the time to prepare the materials will keep this *Express* intervention focused, efficient, and impactful. Providers can draw or print simple faces reflecting common feelings. The faces can then be glued, one per side, to a 4 × 4 × 4 cube. Having this cube ready, the provider will be prepared to present the intervention when a child who would benefit from it presents in the office. This technique can be helpful with children experiencing other concerns besides anger, so having it on hand is quite useful. Check out what the therapist could say below, including a tip for using a die and HQ Card 4.3 rather than a cube.

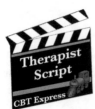

What the Therapist Can Say

"Sometimes angry feelings take over when we first have another feeling. I want to show you a game that will help us practice talking about feelings. Roll the dice and see what feeling face you get. Then we will play a game using the dice."

What the Therapist Can Do

Having the cube ready saves time, or the provider can use a die and HQ Card 4.3. The provider encourages the child to roll the cube or alternatively a die, and then has the child try to name the feeling that is displayed (or corresponds to the number on the die). The provider, child, and any caregivers who are present take turns rolling, naming the feelings, and sharing a time they had that feeling or noticed that feeling in someone else. When the blank face is rolled (e.g., "six" on HQ Card 4.3), the person makes a facial expression of his or her choice and then the other players have to guess what the feeling is.

This *Express* intervention was used with Sierra during a visit attended by her and her mother.

MOM: We are really struggling with Sierra's anger. She blows up at us so easily.

THERAPIST: What kinds of things seem to set her off?

MOM: The other day we were leaving to go out, and we had a new sitter. She completely melted down. We have left her with sitters tons of times and she does fine, but this time she started yelling at me that I wasn't going and she even threw some of her toys.

THERAPIST: Sierra, how were you feeling when it was time for your mom to leave you with the sitter?

SIERRA: I don't know. Bad.

THERAPIST: You felt bad. What kind of bad was it? Did it feel more sad, mad, or scared?

SIERRA: I don't know (*raising her voice*)!

THERAPIST: It seems like just talking about it feels bad. I have an idea. Let's play a game. I have this cube—it is like a die you may use in other games. You roll it and see which face you get.

SIERRA: (*Rolls the die.*)

THERAPIST: Great, what face does that look like to you?

SIERRA: Sad.

THERAPIST: I agree. What is something that might make someone sad?

SIERRA: If their dog ran away.

THERAPIST: That is sad. OK, Mom's turn to roll.

MOM: I got a nervous or scared face.

THERAPIST: What is something that might make someone nervous or scared?

MOM: A really bad storm.

SIERRA: Especially if there is really loud thunder!

THERAPIST: Great job naming those feelings, both of you. Now, Sierra, what is a time you felt nervous or scared?

Depending on the child's skill level and comfort, you may have to work up to more personalized examples by the child. He or she may need to start with identifying feelings other people might have or feeling examples that he or she has observed in others. Once comfortable with those steps, you can work on the child expressing more examples from his or her own life. Here are a few ideas for wording the questions:

"What is something that might make someone feel _____?"

"Tell about a time you noticed someone else was _____."

"What is something that might make you feel _____?"

"Tell about a time you felt _____."

Best Guess

Ages: 6 years and older.

Module: Cognitive Restructuring.

Purpose: Increase the child's ability to take the perspective of others and to cast doubt on the automatic negative thoughts he or she has when interacting with others.

Rationale: Children who struggle with anger often assume a negative intent by others. Best Guess prompts children to consider alternative, less malicious intentions by others.

Materials: HQ Card 4.4a and 4.4b, Best Guess sample and blank card (pp. 75–76), and a writing utensil.

Expected time needed: 10 minutes.

Anger reactions triggered by the belief that one was wronged or judged by someone else can be difficult to identify. Children often don't share or may not be aware of what was going through their mind before the outburst. This was the case with 9-year-old Olivia, who was suspended from school just prior to being seen in a clinic by her primary care physician.

Mom's description of what happened seemed to indicate an escalating pattern of anger and acting-out behaviors, possibly following Olivia feeling as though she was being judged. During the first week of school, Olivia back talked a teacher and was reprimanded. When the teacher walked away, Olivia shoved a peer and claimed the peer had been laughing at her. She was sent home early that day. When she returned to school the next day, several peers asked where she was the day before. Olivia became more agitated and explosive when her peers noticed she had left school, and following this outburst she was again sent home, this time for the rest of the week.

Olivia's immediate reaction seemed to be that others were making fun of or judging her, and thus she lashed out verbally and physically, getting herself in more trouble. Her mother had been focusing on the behaviors (aggression and back talking) but hadn't addressed the trigger for those behaviors, which was Olivia's interpretation of others' behaviors and negative guesses about what they were thinking of her.

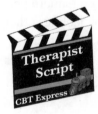

What the Therapist Can Say

THERAPIST: It sounds like it was a rough first week of school.

OLIVIA: The kids there are just mean. When I go back, if they make fun of me again I will punch them in the face.

THERAPIST: It sounds like when the kids ask about where you have been, that makes you very angry.

OLIVIA: Yeah, because they are teasing me for being sent home.

THERAPIST: Possibly, or there could be other reasons they are asking.

OLIVIA: What do you mean?

THERAPIST: Well, did they say why they were asking?

OLIVIA: No.

THERAPIST: Then maybe you made your *best guess* about why they asked, but maybe your first *best guess* was wrong. Let's use this worksheet to see if there is another guess about why they asked where you were.

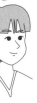

What the Therapist Can Do

The therapist then works with the family to complete HQ Card 4.4. Identifying alternative explanations helps Olivia see that her best guess may not be the only possibility. Youth are typically utterly convinced they've generated the correct interpretation of the situation. When using the Best Guess HQ Card, prompt the child to identify other *possible* interpretations, not necessarily the "right" ones. This early movement toward flexible thinking facilitates future awareness of alternative explanations. This exercise can also lead to discussions about motives and perceptions as well as role plays (see Dress Rehearsal, later in this chapter) for how to handle similar situations in the future. Behavioral practices give children a chance to further rehearse coping strategies. Specifically for Olivia, this next step was key. She was supposed to return to school the following Monday, and was likely to be asked again where she had been.

It Ain't Necessarily So!

Ages: 8 years and older.

Module: Cognitive restructuring.

Purpose: Decrease cognitive rigidity and increase capacity to consider multiple alternatives (reattribution).

Rationale: Angry and aggressive youth tend to judge events as unfair, hostile provocations, and violations of personal rules.

Materials: HQ Cards 4.5a and 4.5b, It Ain't Necessarily So! sample and blank cards (pp. 77–78), and a writing utensil.

Expected time needed: 10 minutes.

Angry and aggressive youth engage in making hostile attributional biases where they arbitrarily misinterpret others' actions as hostile provocations (Dodge, 2006). Moreover, they perceive things that don't go their way as being unfair. It Ain't Necessarily So! is a simple cognitive restructuring intervention that takes its name from a classic song by George and Ira Gershwin and helps young patients think outside their anger-governed mental box.

It Ain't Necessarily So! is very simple to implement. First, the therapist and patient list the angry thought in the left-hand column. Then the patient fills in the blank space that follows "It ain't necessarily so" in the right-hand column. The sample worksheet is a model that shows the patient how to fill in the blank spaces.

What the Therapist Can Say

The following dialogue demonstrates how therapists can introduce and quickly utilize this Express strategy with Esther, who is struggling with anger expression.

THERAPIST: Esther, remember we talked about how when you are angry, you think it is certain that others are purposefully being unfair or testing you to see if you can defend yourself and you feel like you have to?

ESTHER: Yeah, I remember.

THERAPIST: Well, I have this quick exercise called "It Ain't Necessarily So!" It helps you search for other ways to see the situation. Are you willing to try it?

ESTHER: I guess so.

THERAPIST: Let's first look at the sample worksheet. Read the angry thought and the "It ain't necessarily so" comeback.

ESTHER: OK, I read them. . . . Now what?

THERAPIST: Did the comebacks have something in common?

ESTHER: Dude . . . Well, duh . . . They all started with "It ain't necessarily so."

THERAPIST: Good eye . . . exactly right! What I want you to try to do is when you have angry thoughts about people being unfair or purposefully trying to get over on you, try to talk back to these thoughts, starting with "It ain't necessarily so." Do you want to try one?

ESTHER: I guess.

THERAPIST: All right, write down an angry thought that went through your mind today at school.

ESTHER: Sure. Anna-Marie is a true b**ch. She tries to get all the boys not to like me and to like her instead. She thinks she is the only one who is hot. She wants me to be less than her. I've got to not let her do that to me.

THERAPIST: That sure is an angry thought. Now try the comeback. It ain't necessarily so . . .

ESTHER: Well, she is a true b**ch. I can tell you that!

THERAPIST: Remember, Esther, try the "It ain't necessarily so." Is she a 100% true b**ch? Didn't you think she was a really good friend a few weeks ago? Wouldn't that mean at some time she had some not so b**chy things about her? So maybe she did you wrong but it ain't necessarily so that she is a 100% true b**ch.

ESTHER: If you put that way . . . OK.

THERAPIST: Now you continue with the rest.

ESTHER: Hmm. It ain't necessarily so she is more than me.

THERAPIST: What does that mean about you *having to* not let her get over on you?

ESTHER: She *should* respect me!!

THERAPIST: True . . . but do you *have* to get her to do that? Can you let up on the pressure to force her?

ESTHER: Maybe.

THERAPIST: Use the It Ain't Necessarily So! tool.

ESTHER: It ain't necessarily so that I have to *make* her respect me.

In this example, the therapist worked with Esther to modify her angry thoughts in real time during the dialogue to prompt and practice the It Ain't Necessarily So! *Express* intervention. Esther initially struggled to apply the technique, but the therapist kept the interaction focused on the strategy and was not sidetracked by Esther's angry comments. In the end, Esther had the experience of modifying her thoughts during this brief interaction with the therapist, which increases the likelihood of Esther using the strategy again in the future.

Jump Back

Ages: 8 years and older.

Module: Cognitive Restructuring.

Purpose: Interrupt impulsive, angry behaviors by having children stop for a brief time and "jump back" to assess the situation rather than immediately reacting or jumping into the situation.

Rationale: Children respond to anger triggers impulsively and quickly. Jump Back provides a visual image and physical reminder for kids to take a moment and think about the situation before responding.

Materials: HQ Card 4.6, Jump Back (p. 79), and a writing utensil.

Expected time needed: 10 minutes.

Intervening or stopping an anger reaction once it starts can be quite a challenge. Anger outbursts typically include impulsivity and less rational thinking. Therefore, in-depth cognitive techniques or trying to reason with youth in those moments will likely end in escalation by the youth and frustration on the part of the caregiver. Jump Back offers a visual image that children can practice picturing at the moment they start to feel angry. Caregivers can quickly prompt the youth when they see the signs of building anger by reminding them of the image or the Jump Back technique.

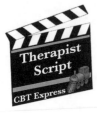

What the Therapist Can Say

"When something happens that is frustrating or makes you angry, your automatic reaction is to just jump right in. If you think someone is being mean to you or telling you something you don't like, you usually get right up in their face, yell, or something like that. But that often ends in you getting in trouble and still not getting what you want.

Rather than jumping in, I want you to picture yourself jumping back, as if someone came around a corner and startled you or you were standing by a road and a car was going by at a high speed. Taking that Jump Back moment and picturing it in your head can give you the moment you need to stop yourself from jumping in and showing your anger in a way that will just end with you getting into more trouble."

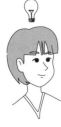

What the Therapist Can Do

First, the provider can role-play with the child, having the child actually physically jump forward and backward to illustrate the concept and help create a more vivid memory of the intervention. Then the child can practice without physically jumping, instead visualizing the jumping in his head. Below is an example of Daniel's school counselor practicing Jump Back with him.

COUNSELOR: It seems like it really bothers you when other kids say something to you during gym or recess.

DANIEL: They are always trying to mess with me when the teachers aren't around.

COUNSELOR: It is hard to stop yourself from jumping in and reacting right away. I noticed you seem to yell at them or shove them as your first response.

DANIEL: They just make me so mad I want to get them.

COUNSELOR: What usually happens next?

DANIEL: Of course the teacher turns around and sees us, so I end up in trouble.

COUNSELOR: I am guessing that makes you even madder.

DANIEL: It is so unfair.

COUNSELOR: What if we try a different strategy? What if instead of jumping in you jump back?

DANIEL: What does that even mean?

COUNSELOR: Good question. Have you ever been startled or surprised by someone walking around a corner unexpectedly?

DANIEL: Sure.

COUNSELOR: And what happened when they suddenly appeared in front of you?

DANIEL: I guess I took a step back because I was surprised or didn't want to crash into them.

COUNSELOR: Exactly. It is like you stepped or jumped back to avoid something bad from happening. We want to do the same thing in your head when someone says something that is frustrating or annoying. Let's practice now. (*Counselor and Daniel stand up.*) Pretend I am a kid in gym who is standing near you waiting for Mrs. Gear to get the class started.

DANIEL: That is exactly when someone would say something like "Move it!"

COUNSELOR: OK, I will be that person. You "jump back" when I say it. "Move it!"

DANIEL: (*Takes a hop backwards.*)

COUNSELOR: What do you notice?

DANIEL: Well, we are further away from each other now, so I can't reach you as easily to shove you.

COUNSELOR: Good point. The Jump Back puts some distance between you and the other kid, and can give you time to think about what to do. You won't always be able to physically jump back, but mentally jumping back can do the same thing. It puts some distance between you and the kid and gives you time to think of what else to do. In this situation, what else could you do?

DANIEL: I guess I could just walk away. Class would be starting soon. Or I could pretend I didn't hear him.

COUNSELOR: Those are great ideas. Let's try it again, but this time instead of physically jumping back, picture yourself doing it in your mind.

The Jump Back strategy helped give Daniel a more concrete experience to picture when he is faced with similar situations at school, while also providing opportunities for further discussions about what situations it is best to Jump Back from. Parents can be included in the discussions, and ideas for home practice should be generated with the families.

I Need to Tell You Something . . .

Ages: Parents of children 6 years and older.

Module: Behavioral Experiments and Exposures.

Purpose: Prompt youth to practice self-regulation strategies before the anger trigger occurs.

Rationale: Children are more likely to be able to engage in newly learned self-regulation strategies when they are calm. Helping them identify coping or self-regulation strategies immediately prior to an anger trigger will increase the likelihood of their using the strategies once the trigger occurs.

Materials: None.

Expected time needed: 5 minutes.

Anger responses are often impulsive reactions to unwanted messages, disappointment, or perceived rejection. Children respond without stopping and thinking, and their behaviors occur before they have considered either the consequences of their behaviors or alternative responses. When emotions are high, problem solving and decision making is more challenging. This *Express* technique helps parents prepare their child for known anger triggers and coaches the child on a more appropriate response, as well as outlines the consequences before the behavior occurs. Consider James, an 8-year-old boy who loses his cool every time his parents tell him "no" or set a limit. His mother describes him as happy and pleasant as long as he is getting his way. Once she sets a limit, he yells, is disrespectful, and sometimes throws objects and slams doors.

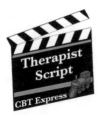

What the Therapist Can Say

"You mentioned that James mostly gets angry when you set a limit, like telling him 'no.' That is called an anger trigger. The good thing is that you know a major trigger for him, so we can try and change the pattern using an intervention called I Need to Tell You Something. . . . This strategy helps prepare James for some disappointing news by reminding him of coping and self-control strategies and then allows you to praise him for use of these strategies, thus focusing your attention on the behaviors you want to see more often. It is kind of like role playing or practicing controlling his anger before the anger kicks in. This can be harder to explain than to show. Let me demonstrate what I mean."

What the Therapist Can Do

The therapist can begin an interaction with the child like the dialogue below. A silly example can be chosen initially to ensure moving through the role play, but then the provider should work to help the family generalize to other situations. Engagement in the discussion and any display of coping or self-regulation strategy by the youth should be praised, and parents can be reminded of the *Praise* parenting block and how to use positive attending during this intervention.

Parents can be reminded to give descriptive positive labels for the desired calm behaviors.

THERAPIST: James, I need to tell you something.

JAMES: (*Looks up from his phone and raises his eyebrows.*)

THERAPIST: Thanks for giving me your attention. I need to tell you something and I need you to practice keeping your voice calm and respectful when I do. If you don't like what I say, let me know calmly.

JAMES: You are acting weird.

THERAPIST: I need you to calmly move from that chair to the one next to it.

JAMES: (*Rolls his eyes and changes chairs.*)

THERAPIST: (*Smiles.*) Thanks—I know that was weird but I appreciate how you just calmly moved chairs. (*to Mom*) If I hadn't told James that I was about to tell him something, what do you think his reaction would have been when I gave him the direction?

MOM: He would have started in with questions, like "Why do you want me to move?"

THERAPIST: OK, so I know this was a silly example, but now let's practice with examples more likely to occur at home.

The therapist then works with the family to identify a specific situation during which this technique could be applied. For James, the family identified an example as being told he can't spend the night at a friend's house.

THERAPIST: You are telling me that James would have trouble controlling his anger at home if you told him he couldn't spend the night at a friend's house. OK, Mom, let's pretend James texted you from school asking if he could spend the night at Kyle's house. You responded that you would talk about it with him after school and he just got home from school.

MOM: OK, let's see. I guess I would start with something like "James, I need to tell you something and I need you to stay calm while we talk."

THERAPIST: Good start, now remember to tell him the good part about staying calm when you also tell him the information that has triggered his anger in the past.

MOM: You asked to stay at Kyle's tonight. You can go to Kyle's tonight if you continue to use your calm voice and respectful words. A sleepover tonight isn't going to work since we have to be up so early tomorrow, but you can stay at Kyle's until 10:30 P.M.

JAMES: (*scowl on his face*) Figures. You don't want to stay up late so I can't spend the night.

THERAPIST: (*Quietly prompts Mom.*) Focus on what he is doing well.

MOM: You are really doing a nice job keeping your voice calm. I know this is disappointing. Next weekend we don't have anywhere to be early Saturday so we can discuss a sleepover for that night.

This may seem overly simplistic to some families, but the few seconds it creates for a "stop and think" response by James can be the difference between a mildly annoyed response (as outlined above in the sample dialogue) and a full-blown anger outburst. Consider how it could have gone *without* the initial preparation or prompt.

MOM: I got your text and sorry but no sleepovers this weekend.

JAMES: *Mom*! Seriously?! You have got to be kidding. Why not?

MOM: Calm down! You are being disrespectful. Do you want to be grounded altogether? You can go for part of the time.

JAMES: Ugh! But that's not fair. What the heck?!?

MOM: Stop yelling!

JAMES: It's so unfair, why can't I go? You never let me do what I want!

MOM: Fine, just stay home then.

JAMES: (*Throws his backpack on the ground, stomps off and slams door.*)

Notice how James and his mother escalate each other with each response. The unexpected nature of the disappointment seems to trigger James from the start. In contrast, the first sample dialogue tells him bad news is coming so he can be prepared and his mom immediately provides reinforcement for self-regulation, as well as distraction by providing information (next weekend he can have a sleepover).

Dress Rehearsal

Ages: 6 years and older.

Module: Behavioral Experiments and Exposures.

Purpose: Practice new ways of responding to identified anger triggers.

Rationale: Reducing the emotional vulnerability to cognitive attributions is only part of the issue. Children must also learn how to respond to potentially ambiguous prompting events and then practice adaptive responses to maximize generalization in daily life.

Materials: None.

Expected time needed: 10–15 minutes.

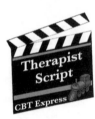

What the Therapist Can Say

"We don't go into opening night of the play having never read the script, practiced the dance moves, or tried on our costume. [*Can adapt to sporting event or academic achievement as applicable to patient's interests.*] When we know an important performance is coming up, we practice, practice, practice. We can practice for times we know we might be angry too. Let's do one practice together now!"

What the Therapist Can Do

After finishing HQ Card 4.4b, Best Guess (pp. 60–61), with Olivia, who was worried that peers would judge her when she was sent home from school, the therapist worked with Olivia and her mother to identify some responses so she could be prepared for the question "Where were you?" It is ideal to prepare two or three options for responding to anger triggers so that children are not overwhelmed with selecting a response, but also do not get stuck when the primary planned reaction is not possible. Once the lines are ready, it's time for the dress rehearsal!

THERAPIST: OK, we've got some ideas for ways you can answer the question "Where were you?" that will hopefully be able to keep you out of trouble. Now we're going to practice them together.

OLIVIA: OK.

THERAPIST: Mom, do you want to be another kid or do you want to be the behind-the-scenes line coach?

MOTHER: I think I will start out by being one of the other kids. I want to see how you do the coaching.

THERAPIST: OK, great. Now, Olivia, when I say "Action," you and your mom are going to pretend like it's your first morning back at school and you're going to practice responding to the other students' questions just like we talked about before. Got it?

OLIVIA: Yeah. This isn't the same, though. I know it's just my mom.

THERAPIST: Sure! We're practicing now when you know it's pretend so that when the real thing happens, you've already done it before. Just like how actresses practice without an audience so they can be great when the audience is sitting watching them.

OLIVIA: I guess that makes sense. Let's do it.

MOTHER: Hey, Olivia! You're back! Where have you been?

OLIVIA: I was at home.

MOTHER: Why weren't you at school?

OLIVIA: (*angrily*) Because you made me get into trouble!

THERAPIST: Ooh, pause! I think we planned a different script, right? Let's try that one again.

MOTHER: Why weren't you at school?

OLIVIA: Are you going to play kickball at lunch?

MOTHER: Yeah, I think so, are you going to play too?

OLIVIA: I think so.

THERAPIST: Great work, Olivia! You did it just like we talked about. The more you practice in these dress rehearsals, the easier it will get when it happens for real.

Olivia and her mom role-played using the new lines in session and then went home and practiced a few times as well. The therapist suggested asking different people to play the other students (e.g., another parent, sibling) so that Olivia could get more rehearsing done. By the time Olivia arrived at school, she was ready to face her anger triggers with the prepared reactions because she had rehearsed her lines to perfection.

Whenever indicated, coach families to use props and/or practice on set to make the rehearsal as realistic as possible. For example, if Olivia had a habit of throwing toys, rehearsals would incorporate Olivia holding something in her hand as she practiced her lines. For children who are more hesitant to approach behavioral practices, it may be helpful to prepare the script in more detail. For example, the youth can either draw out the planned response in a comic format or write it out in a narrative form. This intervention is easily tailored to fit individual patients' hobbies, and the interactive nature engages patients in therapeutic tasks.

Minute-to-Win-It Games

Similar to most other childhood problems, coping with anger and irritation is best accomplished through action. Therefore, experiential exercises that are emotionally evocative are essential (Friedberg & McClure, 2015; Friedberg et al., 2009). Fortunately, there are many ways to give young patients practice dealing with irritating circumstances. Minute-to-win-it exercises fill the bill nicely. There are multiple exercises that can be found online (*http://community.today.com/parentingteam/post/25-minute-to-win-it-games-for-teens-ton-of-fun-guaranteed*; *www.thechaosandtheclutter.com/archives/dollar-store-minute-to-win-it*). However, in this section, we explain three irritating minute-to-win-it games that have therapeutic value.

Frustration Exercises (Ponginator, Breakfast Scramble, Speed Eraser)

Ages: 5 years and older.

Module: Behavioral Experiments and Exposures.

Purpose: Provide practice in adaptive coping with angry emotions and irritating situations.

Rationale: Young patients need to learn and apply their coping skills for anger in emotionally salient contexts. This facilitates proper transfer of learning and the development of genuine self-efficacy.

Materials: See each example below.

Expected time needed: 10–15 minutes.

Ponginator

Website: *www.thechaosandtheclutter.com/archives/dollar-store-minute-to-win-it*

Materials: Empty egg carton, ping pong balls, timer.

The goal of Ponginator is to bounce ping pong balls into an empty egg carton so eight balls stay in the carton within 1 minute. The game is frustrating because you have to find the correct angle to the carton and the ball has to stay within the egg slot.

Breakfast Scramble

Website: *www.thechaosandtheclutter.com/archives/dollar-store-minute-to-win-it*

Materials: Front of a cereal box cut up into 8 or 16 pieces; timer.

To set up for Breakfast Scramble, you will need to cut the front of a cereal box into pieces. Depending on the size of the cereal box and the age of the people participating in your minute-to-win-it challenge, you can cut the box into either 8 or 16 pieces. The goal of the game is to reassemble the puzzle within a minute.

Speed Eraser

Website: *http://community.today.com/parentingteam/post/25-minute-to-win-it-games-for-teens-ton-of-fun-guaranteed*

Materials: Unsharpened pencils with erasers; ceramic cup; timer.

Speed Eraser is a difficult task that prompts lots of frustration. Patients have to bounce the pencil off a hard desktop surface by its eraser so it lands in the ceramic cup. The patient has to land seven pencils in the cup in 1 minute.

What the Therapist Can Do

Remember, the focus of behavioral experimentation is experiencing distress and learning to do something different when encountering the stressor. The therapist should be alert to emotionally provocative moments when the young patient is engaging in the game. When patients appear to get frustrated or irritated, the therapist should ask what the child is feeling and scale it ("On a scale of 1–10, how irritated are you feeling?"). Then, try to capture their thoughts ("What is going through your mind right now?") and coach them through some cognitive restructuring. When the patient completes the experiment, the therapist and patient debrief the task and write down the lessons learned.

Conclusion

Anger and the associated behaviors are common concerns in providers' interactions with families. Triggers for anger outbursts can be many, and treatment may need to be more intense for some youth. However, quick introductions to the *Express* strategies outlined in this chapter can help families begin to manage the anger symptoms, give families hope that something can be done to improve the child's behavior and self-regulation, and engage the child in interventions that set the stage for future sessions. As with many of the other *Express* interventions in this book, the importance of modeling, caregiver involvement, and purposeful use of the short time you have with families are all keys to successful *Express* interventions.

Double Dribble

Do you know how to dribble a basketball? What do you have to do if you are dribbling and then stop dribbling? That's right, you have to do something different than dribbling. You can pass the ball to a teammate, or try to shoot a basket. Dribbling again is against the rules and will result in a "double dribble" call, and the other team will get the ball. Your anger reactions are kind of like a double dribble. You can keep doing the same thing you have always done, but it doesn't end well. Or you can try something different, like passing the ball or taking a shot at the basket. We want to try and do something different with your anger. Instead of dribbling again, we want to try something else. Practice naming other things you can do instead of "double dribbling" when you feel angry.

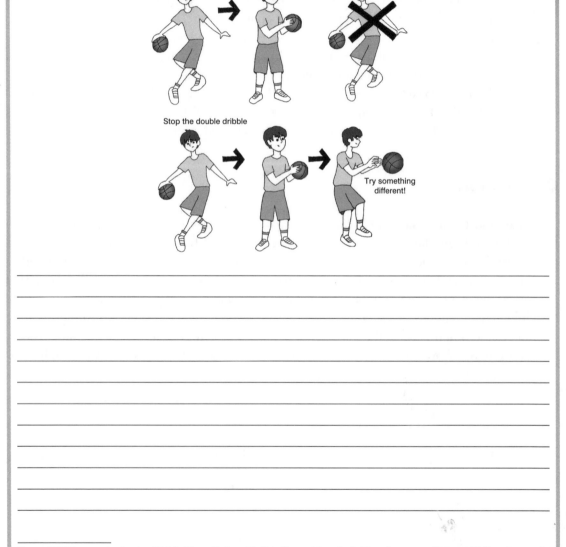

_____

_____

_____

_____

_____

_____

_____

_____

_____

_____

_____

Assertive Anger

What to do when I'm feeling angry:

"I'm feeling . . ." (circle one)

Angry	Mad	Frustrated	Like I'm going to explode
Annoyed	Irritated	Grrrrrr!!	Like I want to scream

I don't like that _____

_____

_____

_____

I really wanted _____

_____

_____

_____

Maybe next time _____

_____

_____

_____

Be sure:

No name calling.   Use kind words.

No blaming.   Use calm voice.

Talk about what you like, want, or need.

Take lots of breaths to keep your body calm when you are talking.

Roll the Dice

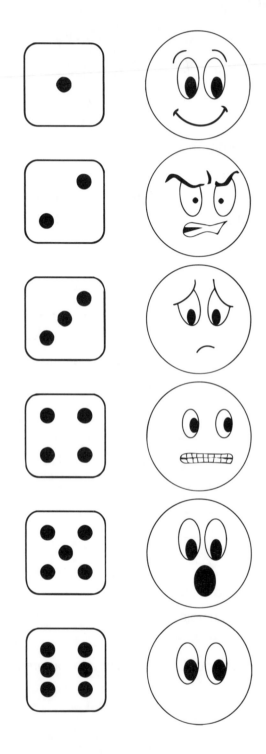

Best Guess: Sample

What happened? Describe the thing that made you mad.

The kids in my class were making fun of me, so I showed them.

What was your guess at the time about what happened?

They were thinking I am stupid and were making fun of me for being sent home from

school the day before.

What are three other things that might have caused that to happen?

1. Sara told them I got sent home and that they should ask me about it.

2. They didn't see what happened and were just wondering where I was.

3. The teacher told them I was suspended and they were trying to find out why.

What is your best guess now about what happened?

They didn't see what happened and were just wondering where I was.

Best Guess

What happened? Describe the thing that made you mad.

_____

_____

_____

_____

What was your guess at the time about what happened?

_____

_____

_____

_____

What are three other things that might have caused that to happen?

1. _____

_____

2. _____

_____

3. _____

_____

What is your best guess now about what happened?

_____

_____

_____

_____

It Ain't Necessarily So!: Sample

	It Ain't Necessarily So! Comeback
Angry Thought	
She salted me when talking about me and my man. She really did me dirty.	**It ain't necessarily so** that she did me dirty like that. She was just talking like a fool.
My father is an unfair SOB.	**It ain't necessarily so** that he is unfair and a SOB. He is just stressed out and messed up.
Rules are made to be broken. I am nobody's puppet.	**It ain't necessarily so** that all rules are made to be broken and that following rules makes me a puppet.
	It ain't necessarily so
	It ain't necessarily so
	It ain't necessarily so
	It ain't necessarily so

It Ain't Necessarily So!

Angry Thought	It Ain't Necessarily So! Comeback
	It ain't necessarily so
	It ain't necessarily so
	It ain't necessarily so
	It ain't necessarily so
	It ain't necessarily so
	It ain't necessarily so
	It ain't necessarily so

Jump Back

Sometimes when something happens, people don't stop to think about what is going on and they just "jump in" and respond. You are working on waiting to respond, or "jumping back," before deciding if jumping in will work best for you. Think of a time you got mad or angry and reacted. What happened when you jumped in right away? What might have happened if you first jumped back and assessed the situation? Use the worksheet below to practice.

Thing that made me mad: _____

_____

_____

How I jumped in: _____

_____

_____

_____

What happened after I jumped in: _____

_____

_____

_____

_____

What might have happened if I jumped back first?:

_____

_____

_____

_____

_____

_____

_____

_____

Emotion Dysregulation

"She completely melts down over nothing—and then it takes forever for her to calm down!"

"I just don't get it—he never seems upset about anything until an explosion."

"We're constantly afraid of what will set her off."

"I never know how she's feeling. No matter what it is, she won't say a thing."

Children with emotion dysregulation are a challenge for parents, teachers, coaches, and providers. Their explosive moods and behaviors are scary and even dangerous at times. Emotion regulation is how children experience and respond to strong feelings (Gross, 1998). It does not come naturally to many of the children we treat, but learning to regulate emotions is a critical developmental process that helps youth function socially, express emotions effectively, and cope with the world around them (Southam-Gerow & Kendall, 2002).

Children differ in the way they experience emotions from the day they are born. We have all observed differences that even biological siblings demonstrate in their expression of emotions. For example, some babies cry easily and are described by parents as "fussy" from day one, while others are described as "always happy," only cry "when they need something," and then are quickly soothed. Extensive research on temperament has demonstrated that these differences can be observed from a very early age and are likely to be relatively stable over time (Beauchaine, Hinshaw & Pang, 2010; Carthy, Horesch, Apter, Edge, & Gross, 2010; Frick & Morris, 2004; Lavigne, Gouze, Hopkins, Bryant, & LeBailly, 2012; Martel, Gremillion, & Roberts, 2012; Muris & Ollendick, 2005; Waldman et al., 2011).

Dispositional vulnerabilities interact with environmental factors to determine emotional meltdowns. In infancy and early childhood, emotion regulation is controlled externally by caregiver influences (Frick & Morris, 2004). Caregivers differ in their responses to children's emotions. Some parents tend to notice and respond more quickly to subtle signals of distress (e.g., a slight grimace), while others may wait to jump in until a stronger display of emotion is present, such as crying. Parents and other caregivers directly and indirectly teach children

roughout childhood. Parental responses to a child's emotional expres-
force or punish those behaviors and contribute to a child's learning
ent–child relationships suggests that there are not a discrete set of
and "bad" parent behaviors in response to emotions; rather it is the
he child's temperament and the parental responses that determines
...up serves adaptive development or contributes to difficulties with emo-
gulation (Chess & Thomas, 1999).

Deficits in emotion regulation are seen in most if not all childhood disorders (Aldao, Nolen-Hoeksema, & Schweizer, 2010). Frequently, challenges with emotion regulation precede the onset of other symptoms, suggesting that emotion dysregulation is a risk factor for psychopathology and not a consequence (McLaughlin, Hatzenbuehler, Mennin, & Nolen-Hoeksema, 2011). Thus, a clinician's efforts to target emotion regulation may yield a preventative benefit in reducing the likelihood of future clinical symptoms in addition to solving the problem with which a family presents. This preventative benefit makes the *CBT Express* interventions presented in this chapter ideal for inclusion in specialty clinics, primary care, schools, and other settings where children and families may be seen for prevention or early intervention.

Throughout this chapter, look for key examples of *CBT Express* scripts and interventions to improve emotion regulation. You will also find references to the Parenting Blocks for Modifying Behavior, first introduced in Chapter 3, at relevant points in this chapter.

Brief Statement Regarding Evidence-Based Treatments

CBT targets emotion regulation both indirectly and directly (Southam-Gerow & Kendall, 2002). Psychoeducation often includes increasing knowledge about emotions, such as the relationship between thoughts and feelings, the benefits of emotions, and behaviors associated with different emotions (Friedberg & Brelsford, 2011; Hannesdottir & Ollendick, 2007). Self-monitoring of emotions increases emotional awareness and facilitates emotional expression (Suveg, Morelen, Brewer, & Thomassin, 2010). Basic behavioral training can include critical emotion regulation strategies, such as problem solving and relaxation. Relaxation reduces the physiological component of emotion (Hannesdottir & Ollendick, 2007), which can interfere with effective use of other strategies, such as problem solving and cognitive restructuring (Suveg et al., 2010). Problem solving can be utilized to identify strategies for coping with emotionally salient situations (Hannesdottir & Ollendick, 2007). Cognitive restructuring is one of the most effective adaptive emotion regulation strategies and is a critical element of CBT interventions for a variety of problems (Friedberg & Brelsford, 2011). Exposures to emotionally evocative situations decrease distress, increase self-efficacy, challenge faulty cognitions, and decrease emotional avoidance (Friedberg et al., 2011).

Additionally, emotion regulation is explicitly targeted in some empirically supported treatment protocols for youth. For example, the Unified Protocol for the Treatment of Emotional Disorders (UP; Allen, Ehrenreich, & Barlow, 2005) addresses a broad range of internalizing symptoms by integrating contemporary learning theory, cognitive neuroscience, and emotion regulation literature. The UP is an efficacious treatment in adults (Allen et al.,

2005) and has been adapted for use with adolescents with promising results (Ehrenreich, Goldstein, Wright, & Barlow, 2009). Similarly, dialectical behavior therapy (DBT; Linehan, 1993) explicitly targets emotion regulation in suicidal individuals by decreasing maladaptive emotion regulation strategies, increasing distress tolerance and emotion regulation skills, and decreasing experiential avoidance. DBT has a substantial body of research supporting its efficacy with adults and has been adapted for adolescents as well (Miller, Rathus, & Linehan, 2006). Southam-Gerow (2016) has compiled an extensive collection of creative emotion regulation interventions for children and adolescents that target emotional awareness, emotion understanding, empathy, and emotion regulation.

Presenting Concerns and Symptoms

Most youth who present with emotional difficulties can be thought of as either *overcontrolled* or *undercontrolled*. Some children try to stuff emotions in proverbial boxes—we call these children overcontrolled. They avoid expressing emotions and rely heavily on pushing away emotional responses in an attempt to regulate their feelings. These children may deny feeling upset despite evidence to the contrary. They may avoid eye contact when displaying even the slightest hint of emotion, and may avoid emotionally salient topics or events. This pattern is illustrated by 9-year-old Raj, whose parents were confused by his behavior. Raj never seemed to be upset, yet at times he would completely shut down, physically freezing in place and refusing to speak.

Undercontrolled youth, on the other hand, wear their emotions on their sleeves. They may be prone to emotional outbursts. These are children who have difficulty controlling their feelings and may express their emotions in inappropriate, ineffective, or destructive ways. At the slightest provocation, 5-year-old Michael was prone to explosive temper tantrums that could last as long as an hour. His parents were desperate for help, explaining that they felt they were constantly "walking on eggshells," trying to avoid an outburst. Both overcontrolled and undercontrolled children tend to have maladaptive beliefs about emotions, need help learning to express and regulate emotions appropriately, and can benefit from brief emotion-focused interventions. Importantly, some children may overcontrol their emotions at some times and in some contexts while undercontrolling their emotions in other situations. Mindy, a 7-year-old girl, avoided emotional experiences and expression at school but frequently displayed out-of-control emotional outbursts at home. Mindy and her family would benefit from *Express* strategies presented in this chapter, which include interventions for both emotion regulation difficulties. Throughout this chapter, you will see the terms *overcontrol* and *undercontrol* next to each intervention to let you know which of the two groups (often both!) would benefit from the intervention.

Interventions with Parents

Parents of overcontrolled and undercontrolled children benefit from psychoeducation about emotions and learning specific emotion-focused skills. Specifically, teaching parents to validate, model, and reinforce appropriate emotion regulation and expression, as well as to avoid reinforcement of dysregulation, are fundamental clinical tasks.

The parenting blocks introduced in Chapter 3 will help form the structure of these interventions. In addition to the basic building blocks you have been using with parents, we are now adding modeling. Modeling is a powerful tool for therapists to use in teaching skills to parents, and then parents can demonstrate/model the use of these skills for their children. Therapists should point out their own modeling and the parents' opportunities for modeling during family interactions.

For each of these parent strategies, the therapist is encouraged to teach the technique, apply the skill by practicing in session with the parent, provide corrective feedback, keep practicing, and troubleshoot how parents can remember to use the skill at home and in times of stress.

The praise and modeling block will be particularly applicable during these interventions. Modeling appropriate emotion regulation will teach children self-regulation skills, and positive attention to the child's use of appropriate emotion regulation will increase the frequency of those desired behaviors in the future. "What the Therapists Can Say" and "What the Therapist Can Do" sections throughout this chapter will help you apply the *Express* strategies while working with families.

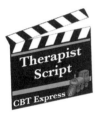

What the Therapist Can Say

"Remember when we talked about building blocks to parenting? How there are key blocks that can be used multiple ways in different situations to help improve your child's behavior and functioning? Well today we are going to use the praise block and the modeling block to help improve your child's self-regulation. These blocks will be stacked together to add to the effectiveness of the interventions."

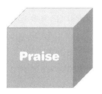 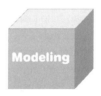

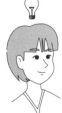

What the Therapist Can Do

This is a great time to pull out the wooden blocks and demonstrate! Use examples from earlier in treatment, such as referring to how the parents used the praise block to increase their child's compliant behavior. Then illustrate how to combine modeling of self-regulation strategies with praise to instances of appropriate self-regulation by the child, while introducing the following skills and interventions.

Facts about Feelings (overcontrol and undercontrol)

Ages: Parents of children of any age; children/teens 10 years and older.

Module: Psychoeducation.

Purpose: Increase parents' understanding of emotions so they can effectively model and reinforce appropriate emotional expression for their children.

Rationale: When parents understand these important facts about feelings, they are better able to recognize their own emotional experiences, teach their children about emotions, and respond effectively to children's emotional expression and behaviors.

Materials: HQ Card 5.1, Facts about Feelings (p. 103).

Expected time needed: 10–15 minutes.

Having a basic understanding of feelings is a critical first step for parents in order to benefit from other emotion regulation strategies. Most interventions that specifically target emotion regulation strategies begin with psychoeducation about emotions that are consistent with the critical facts listed below (Linehan, 2014; Ehrenreich, Goldstein, Wright, & Barlow, 2009; Southam-Gerow, 2016). Several take-away messages for parents are essential. They include:

1. Feelings are important.
2. Feelings are not always accurate.
3. Feelings have different components.
4. Feelings can have different intensities.
5. Feelings do not last forever.

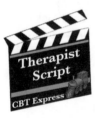

What the Therapist Can Say

"Sometimes when emotions are intense, feel out of control, or are getting in the way, it can seem like feelings themselves are the problem. Learning some facts about feelings can help clarify the problem because the truth is, feelings are really important and we definitely don't want to get rid of them. In fact, not having feelings would lead to a whole lot of other even bigger problems! If we are going to tackle some of the problems your child is facing with emotions, we want to make sure we really understand them. That's why we start off learning these Facts about Feelings."

What the Therapist Can Do

Facts about Feelings should be reviewed with parents to be sure they have a solid understanding of these aspects of emotions. They should also be reviewed with youth ages 10 years and older. HQ Card 5.1 can be introduced in the visit and taken home by families to reinforce the use of this *Express* intervention.

Take the following example of 12-year-old Delilah and her mother.

THERAPIST: I understand that you're concerned about how Delilah handles her emotions.

MOM: She is so sensitive! It's like every day there's some new meltdown, and they can last hours! I just don't know what to do anymore.

THERAPIST: That must be really frustrating for you—and Delilah, I bet it's not fun for you either!

DELILAH: (*Pouts.*) It's not.

THERAPIST: Well, we are going to work together to help both of you understand emotions better and learn new ways to deal with them. How does that sound?

DELILAH: OK, I guess.

THERAPIST: Did you know that feelings are actually super important and we have them for a reason? For example, if you were on a walk in the park and you saw a bear growling at you, how would you feel?

MOM: Pretty scared.

THERAPIST: Absolutely! And it's a good thing you'd feel scared, because that bear is dangerous and you need to make sure you get yourself to a safe place. Fear tells us that we might be in danger and helps us prepare to escape or protect ourselves. Other emotions can help us too. For example, anger tells us something is unfair and can prepare us to fight or defend ourselves. And sadness lets us know that we lost something important and helps other people know that we need support. These are just a few examples of how emotions help us out—and that's why we don't want to get rid of emotions. We want to learn new ways to cope with them so we don't get so overwhelmed.

This dialogue illustrates how to introduce and begin teaching a family the Facts about Feelings. The therapist made sure to engage both Delilah and her mother, use age-appropriate examples, and provide a rationale for emotion-related interventions.

After introducing this concept to families, remember to cover all five key facts to make sure families have a solid understanding of emotions (see Figure 5.1). Reviewing these concepts with parents and children together allows you to make sure all family members have the same basic understanding. Although some of the emotion regulation strategies for youth are effective even if this baseline knowledge is not there, helping parents understand emotions enables them to act as effective emotion coaches and serves as a foundation for the following *Express* interventions.

---

1. Feelings are important and beneficial.
   a. Fear helps us know if we are in danger.
   b. Anger helps us prepare for a fight.
   c. Sadness tells us we lost something important and helps others know we need support.
2. Feelings aren't always accurate.
   d. Sometimes we are afraid of things that aren't dangerous.
   e. Sometimes we feel angry or sad because of what we THINK someone meant, and it turns out they meant something different.
3. Feelings have different components: thoughts, body sensations, behaviors.
4. Feelings have different intensities—for example, 0–10, 0–100.
5. Feelings don't last forever.

FIGURE 5.1. Facts about Feelings: Summary.

Validate Emotions: Is This Valid?; No "Buts" Allowed (overcontrol and undercontrol)

Ages: Parents of children of all ages.

Module: Psychoeducation; Basic Behavioral Tasks.

Purpose: Teach parents to validate their children's emotions.

Rationale: When parents learn to validate children's emotions using behavioral rehearsal and corrective feedback, they communicate that emotions are acceptable and make sense, they increase children's adaptive emotional expression, and decrease maladaptive regulation techniques.

Materials: HQ Cards 5.2, Is This Valid?: Parental Validation Practice (p. 104), and 5.3, No "Buts" Allowed (p. 105).

Expected time needed: 10–15 minutes.

Validation communicates to children that their parents understand their perspective. Children look to their parents to understand their own experiences. When parents validate emotions, they help their child increase awareness and understanding of emotions, as well as communicate the message that emotions are a normal part of life. This is critical for both children who overcontrol and undercontrol their emotions. For overcontrolled children, it is important for parents to communicate that emotions are acceptable and that emotional expression is normal and understandable. Validation of emotion for overcontrolled children helps to increase their emotional expression and reduce their use of expressive suppression. Children who are undercontrolled benefit from parents who communicate these same messages. This type of validation serves to decrease emotional arousal in undercontrolled youth and to increase use of regulation strategies.

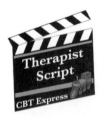

What the Therapist Can Say

"Communicating that you understand your child's emotion can help her to calm down. Instead of saying, 'don't be upset' or 'it's not a big deal,' validate your child's emotion by letting her know you see her perspective. Validation means communicating to your child that her experience makes sense to you. You could say, 'I can tell that you're really upset' or 'It makes sense to feel sad when someone hurts your feelings.' Even if you don't understand or agree with how she is responding to her feelings, you can still validate the feeling. If your child threw a tantrum and broke a toy, you can still validate her emotion ('you must have been really frustrated') without telling her it's OK to behave that way. By validating emotions, you help your child recognize her own emotions, and accept that emotions are OK and make sense."

What the Therapist Can Do

It is essential that you not only explain validation but also have parents practice in session. They may seem to understand the concept but struggle to apply it accurately. By practicing in session, you have the opportunity to give corrective feedback, which will increase the chances of parents validating effectively at home. When practicing, use examples that are relevant to the particular child and that come from real encounters between the parent and child. Refer to HQ Card 5.2 for more practice examples for parents.

Next, encourage parents to avoid using "but." This often turns what started out as a validating statement into an invalidating one. For example, if a parent says, "I understand you are feeling sad, *but* it'll all blow over tomorrow," the validating first half will be forgotten and the child will remember the well-intentioned yet invalidating second half. See HQ Card 5.3 for additional examples that give parents opportunities for practice.

Here's an example of practicing validation with Mrs. Miller, whose 10-year-old son, Anthony, has been irritable and displaying emotional outbursts. In other words, Anthony is undercontrolling his emotions.

THERAPIST: We've been talking about how to validate Anthony's emotions. Let's practice: I'll be Anthony and I want you to practice validation.

MRS. MILLER: OK.

THERAPIST: (*as Anthony*) I had the worst day at school today! Everyone is so mean to me—I'm never going back!

MRS. MILLER: I can tell you're really upset, but they probably weren't really being mean to you, it just seemed that way.

THERAPIST: Great job reflecting the emotion when you said, "I can tell you're really upset." I know you were trying to make Anthony feel better by saying his friends probably weren't trying to be mean. Remember that we want to communicate that we understand how he feels and not try to change it yet. How do you think you could change that second part to be more validating?

MRS. MILLER: Hmm, what if I said, "No one likes when people are mean to them."?

THERAPIST: That's a great validation! You're showing him that you understand how he feels and that it makes sense given the circumstances.

This dialogue illustrates the importance of not only teaching about validation but actually practicing with parents. As with most new skills, parents benefit from rehearsal in session, corrective feedback, and repeated practice in order to achieve mastery. The therapist modeled providing specific praise, giving corrective feedback in a gentle yet straightforward manner, and reviewing the rationale for validation. It is also critical to teach validation to parents of overcontrolled youth. Here is an example of practicing validation with Mr. Berry, the father of 12-year-old Sonja, who has difficulty expressing her emotions.

THERAPIST: Let's say Sonja gets home from school, drops her backpack on the ground, and sits on the couch pouting. How would you have responded to that before?

MR. BERRY: I would say, don't drop your stuff on the floor! Go put it away and knock it off with that attitude!

THERAPIST: Now having learned about validation and how important it is, what could you say instead that would tell her you understand how she feels?

MR. BERRY: Hmm, I really don't know.

THERAPIST: How do you think Sonja might be feeling?

MR. BERRY: Upset maybe?

THERAPIST: Seems like it. What if you said, "You seem upset."?

MR. BERRY: I guess I could do that. Do you really think that'll help?

THERAPIST: Let's give it a try and see if it does.

Some parents benefit from being given specific language to use when validating. This dialogue illustrates teaching validation with a parent who has a hard time identifying validating responses to his daughter. The therapist can suggest phrases to start with, then have the parent practice to increase comfort and confidence.

Do as I Say, and as I Do! (overcontrol and undercontrol)

Ages: Parents of children of all ages.

Module: Basic Behavioral Tasks.

Purpose: Teach parents to model adaptive emotional expression and regulation for their children.

Rationale: Watching others is one of the most important ways children learn, and children will watch and learn whether parents express and regulate emotions in a healthy or unhealthy way. Parents can learn to impact their children's emotional behaviors by intentionally modeling adaptive emotional expression and regulation.

Materials: None.

Expected time needed: 5–10 minutes.

By observing their parents, children learn acceptable ways to express emotions. If parents do not feel that any emotional expression is acceptable, children are likely to hold similar views or feel shame when they express emotions. Although parents typically understand that children often learn by mimicking what they observe in others, they may not recognize that they provide a model for emotion expression just like other behaviors. Overcontrolled and undercontrolled children benefit from parents who show their emotions in appropriate ways. Parents of overcontrolled children may need to focus on expressing their emotions more often so children see that showing emotions is acceptable. Parents of undercontrolled children should be cautious about modeling emotion dysregulation and strive to model moderate levels of emotional expression.

Similarly, children learn strategies for regulating emotions by observing the way in which parents respond to emotions. If parents are seen suppressing emotions, avoiding emotional experiences, behaving destructively, or using substances to regulate emotions, children may learn these maladaptive emotion regulation strategies as well. Parents benefit from learning the same emotion regulation strategies that are being taught to their child, both in order to act as a coach and supporter in the home as well as to model these skills themselves.

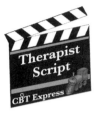

What the Therapist Can Say

"I'm sure you can think of times when your child copied something you were doing or saying—whether you wanted them to or not! This can be really adorable and helpful, like a child wanting his own broom to sweep the floor just like Daddy does. It can also be frustrating or embarrassing, like a child repeating a swear word in public that she overheard you say when you stubbed your toe. This tendency of kids to mimic their parents is just as important when it comes to showing emotions and coping with them. The way you express your feelings and how you manage emotions teaches your children what to do. By modeling the types of emotional expression and emotion regulation that you want to see in your child, you can help him or her learn these important skills."

What the Therapist Can Do

The fact that children copy their parents is the reason it is essential to teach parents the same skills you want their children to learn. Seven-year-old Guillermo would shut down and stop talking when overwhelmed. His parents reported that they expressed their emotions to each other but felt it was best to keep that private and did not talk about or display emotions in front of their son. For example, when stressed about work, Guillermo's father would come home, eat dinner alone in his office, and then watch TV without talking to his wife or son until bedtime. In session the therapist worked with Guillermo's father having him practice saying, "I'm stressed from work and need some time to myself. I'm going to eat in the office tonight so I can get more work done." Although he still withdrew from the family when emotionally overwhelmed, by labeling his emotion and explaining his behavior, he modeled for Guillermo that it is OK to feel overwhelmed and take a break when needed.

The Praise building block introduced in Chapter 3 is a powerful tool for parents reinforcing appropriate expressions of emotion, and therapists can use the block to illustrate the impact of praise during this intervention. Therapists should encourage parents to use the Praise block while practicing this intervention, and can pair it with the modeling block for these interactions.

The therapist also practiced modeling and labeling adaptive emotion regulation with Guillermo's mother. In fact, she had already been engaging in deep breathing as an adaptive coping strategy, but she typically went into another room away from Guillermo to do so. After learning about modeling emotion regulation, she began telling Guillermo, "I need to take some deep breaths. Will you do them with me?" This served not only to illustrate effective emotion regulation, but also encouraged Guillermo to practice deep breathing, which he enjoyed because it was a special thing he did with his mother.

Amp Up Expression (overcontrol and undercontrol)

Ages: Parents of children of all ages.

Module: Basic Behavioral Tasks.

Purpose: Teach parents to use behavioral principles like positive reinforcement to increase adaptive emotion expression.

Rationale: Just like any other behavior, emotional expression responds well to reinforcement. If parents positively reinforce adaptive emotional expression, children will engage in these behaviors more frequently. Teaching parents to apply basic behavioral principles to their children's emotional behaviors will help them shape the behaviors they want.

Materials: HQ Card 5.4, Amp Up Expression (p. 106), and a writing utensil.

Expected time needed: 5–10 minutes.

As with any behavior a parent wants to increase, reinforcing appropriate expressions of emotion will increase this behavior in youth. It is critical to notice adaptive expressions of emotion because if these behaviors are ignored, overcontrolled children are less likely to express emotions in the future while undercontrolled children are likely to escalate their emotional expression and become dysregulated. Appropriate expressions of emotion can be reinforced in a variety of ways, with attention being the most important reinforcer. Attention in the form of praise, comfort, nurturing, or assistance is a good choice for parents of both over and undercontrolled youth. As with any reinforcement strategy, choosing a reinforcer that is potent for a particular child is critical. Work with parents to complete the HQ Card 5.4 for "amping up" and reinforcing appropriate emotional expression and regulation.

See Chapter 2 (HQ Card 2.3) for what to say and do when teaching parents reinforcement. The same behavioral principles apply for increasing emotion-related behaviors.

Sometimes it can be difficult to determine whether a particular child's emotional expression is overcontrolled, appropriate, or undercontrolled. The following chart describes behavior one might observe for a variety of emotions and can be used to identify whether a child is struggling with overcontrol, undercontrol, or both.

	Overcontrolled	Appropriate	Undercontrolled
Sad	Refuses to talk about feeling; will not cry (especially in front of others)	Tearful, crying; seeks comfort from others; able to be soothed	Sobbing for hours; screaming; throwing self on the floor; inconsolable; may threaten to harm self
Angry	Fuming; refuses to talk; may stomp around but avoids confrontation	Raises voice, may yell; expresses anger/frustration; looks for solutions	Destruction of property; aggressive toward others; screaming/yelling; kicking, hitting
Scared	Freezes; refuses to talk; avoids feared situation; may become pale/cold; reports headaches, stomachaches, or other physical symptoms	Some physiological symptoms (e.g., shaking, tearful); hesitant about approaching; seeks help or protection; able to be coaxed to face fear	Panicked; intense physiological symptoms (e.g., hyperventilating, sweating); may scream/cry; may throw up
Happy	Reluctant or unable to engage in activity; minimal expression of positive emotions; limited engagement with others; behavior is underactive for situation (e.g., sitting quietly while peers are cheering at a sporting event)	Smiles; expresses excitement/anticipation/joy; joins in activities; explores; behavior is appropriate to situation (e.g., running around while playing tag with friends); shares with peers or parents	Overexcited; may have difficulty engaging in activity; behavior is overactive for situation (e.g., screaming in excitement in a library); difficulty engaging with others due to enthusiasm

It can be challenging to reinforce appropriate responses. The following chart offers some ideas of how to validate, praise, and give attention as a reward for adaptive expressions of various emotions.

	Validation	Praise		Attention
		Overcontrolled	**Undercontrolled**	
Sad	"I can tell you are really sad right now."	"Thank you for letting me know how you feel."	"I am really proud of you for expressing your sadness this way."	Offer a hug, sit together
Angry	"It makes sense to be angry about this!"	"I'm so glad to know you are feeling this way."	"You are doing such a good job staying calm even though you are really angry."	Walk around together
Scared	"You must be so scared."	"You are so brave for talking about this."	"I can tell that you are working really hard on facing your fears."	Offer a hug, sit together
Happy	"You seem like you are having a lot of fun!"	"I love seeing how excited you are."	"Great job participating in the game!"	Give a high-5

Reinforcing Effective Emotion Regulation: Catch Them Using Skills; Reward Chart (overcontrol, undercontrol)

Ages: Parents of youth of all ages.

Module: Basic Behavioral Tasks.

Purpose: Teach parents to use behavioral principles like positive reinforcement to increase adaptive emotion regulation.

Rationale: Just like any other behavior, expression regulation responds well to reinforcement. If parents positively reinforce adaptive emotion regulation, children will engage in these behaviors more frequently. Teaching parents to apply basic behavioral principles to their children's emotional behaviors will help them shape the behaviors they want.

Materials: HQ Cards 5.5, Catch Them Using Skills (p. 107), 5.6a and 5.6b, Reward Chart sample and blank cards (pp. 108–109), and a writing utensil.

Expected time needed: 5–10 minutes.

Adaptive emotion regulation can be increased in youth through parental reinforcement. Both overcontrolled and undercontrolled youth likely struggle to regulate emotions in an effective way. Overcontrolled children rely heavily on expressive suppression, so parents should be looking for and reinforcing alternative emotion regulation strategies, such as those described later in this chapter in the section "Interventions with Children and Adolescents." Undercontrolled children may lack effective strategies or utilize maladaptive strategies such as aggressive behavior, self-injurious behavior, or substance use. Parents of these children should similarly be on the lookout for moments of effective regulation (e.g., taking deep breaths, using a relaxation technique, distraction) and provide reinforcement. With both emotional expression and emotion regulation, attention is the key reinforcer. Praise, comfort, nurturing, and assistance are excellent choices.

Priya, a 10-year-old with undercontrolled emotions, was learning new emotion regulation strategies and did a great job practicing them in session. Her parents were frustrated that she rarely seemed to use these new skills at home. This was a perfect time to focus on positive reinforcement. As a family, they picked two of Priya's favorite emotion regulation skills—deep breathing and playing with her dog. Priya's parents practiced noticing and praising their daughter's emotion regulation. Priya's mother felt most comfortable using verbal praise and came up with these examples: "Great job with your deep breathing!"; "I love how you took Toto [the dog] outside to play when you got frustrated"; and "Wow, I can tell that deep breathing really helped calm you down." Priya's father had a harder time with verbal praise and felt more comfortable with physical expressions. He started out giving Priya a high-5 anytime he noticed her using an emotion regulation skill, and later he and Priya came up with a special fist bump. They also made a chart where Priya got a star each time she practiced a skill and agreed that when she earned 15 stars, she could pick a movie to watch together as a family. HQ Cards 5.5, 5.6a, and 5.6b will guide providers in using these interventions with families.

Don't Throw Fuel on the Fire! (undercontrol)

Ages: Parents of youth of all ages.

Module: Basic Behavioral Tasks.

Purpose: Teach parents to extinguish behaviors and tolerate the extinction burst.

Rationale: Parents of undercontrolled youth are often unintentionally reinforcing behaviors they want to decrease—this is like pouring on lighter fluid when you think you're using the fire extinguisher. In order to extinguish these behaviors, it is essential to remove reinforcement for maladaptive emotional expression and regulation.

Materials: HQ Card 5.7, Don't Throw Fuel on the Fire (pp. 110–111), and a writing utensil.

Expected time needed: 10–15 minutes.

Often undercontrolled children develop a pattern of emotion dysregulation in part due to unintentional reinforcement of the behaviors. For example, 4-year-old Tyler often threw a tantrum when told "no." When Tyler had an emotional outburst in a public place, such as a grocery store, his parents were so embarrassed that they often gave in and got him the candy or toy they had originally denied. By giving in to Tyler's request following his display of emotion dysregulation, his parents were positively reinforcing this inappropriate behavior. It is important to remember that children generally find attention from parents to be rewarding, even if parents view it as "negative attention" or a type of punishment. Lecturing is a good example of this. Although parents often see lectures as a punishment, some children are reinforced by this one-on-one attention from a parent. This attention will add fuel to the fire instead of putting it out.

Whenever 11-year-old Lillian got angry and broke one of her sister's toys, her parents would lecture her for up to 30 minutes. Although her parents viewed this as punishing, they noticed that Lillian was breaking toys more and more often. This tells us that Lillian was being reinforced by the one-on-one time with Mom or Dad. The first step is to immediately and consistently discontinue any reinforcement of maladaptive emotional expressions or regulation. Instead, parents should be coached to ignore dysregulated behavior while enthusiastically reinforcing adaptive behavior. Lillian's parents were coached to notice when she expressed anger without breaking toys (e.g., "I see you are getting frustrated, and I like how you are keeping your hands to yourself") and to implement a brief time-out from playtime and extra chores instead of lecturing after Lillian broke a toy. See HQ Card 5.7 for more information about breaking this cycle.

Beware the Extinction Burst!

When parents have been consistently or intermittently reinforcing emotion dysregulation, it is critical for them to halt this process if they hope to help their child regulate his emotions appropriately. However, when parents stop reinforcing dysregulated behavior, children will predictably escalate the behavior in an attempt to receive reinforcement. This is called an extinction burst, and it occurs whenever reinforcement is abruptly withdrawn (Cooper, Heron, & Heward, 1987). For parents who are trying to extinguish a behavior, persisting through the extinction burst is often the most difficult time. It is important to prepare parents for this pattern and encourage them to view the temporary worsening of behavior as a sign they are on the path to extinction. This can help them stick with the plan instead of giving in to more extreme behavior.

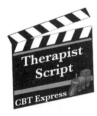

What the Therapist Can Say

"You have been doing a great job learning these new ways to change your child's behavior and it sounds like you are ready to start ignoring his whining and reinforcing 'big-kid talk.' Now, before you go home and get started, I need to warn you about the extinction burst. When parents have been giving a lot of attention for whining and all of a sudden they stop, kids often escalate the behavior to try to get that attention. This is called the extinction burst and it can trip up some parents, but since you're going to know what to look for, you will be able to get through it. The key to surviving the extinction burst is to know it's coming and stick with the program. Maybe he takes the whining up to level 10 or even level 100, maybe he starts yelling, or stomping his feet. Remind yourself that this is the extinction burst and stick with the program. That means 100% ignoring until he uses his 'big-kid voice.'"

What the Therapist Can Do

Keep an eye out for opportunities to point out unintentional reinforcement and the extinction burst in session. For example, you might notice that while you're reviewing homework with Tyrell's father, 6-year-old Tyrell starts tugging on his father's sleeve and whining, "Dad, I'm hungry. Dad, I need a snack. Dad? Dad?? Dad???" until Tyrell's dad yells "WHAT?? Can't you see I'm talking to the doctor??"

This is a great opportunity to walk Tyrell's father through the key elements of this behavioral intervention. You can praise his initial attempts at ignoring Tyrell's whining and validate his frustration with Tyrell's escalating behavior. By pointing out that this was an extinction burst, Tyrell's father will be more able to identify similar situations at home. Finally, you can have Tyrell and his father re-create the scene and practice a new way of responding. You can even switch roles (e.g., have Tyrell play Dad and you play Tyrell) to keep it fun.

In-session examples like this can take these skills to the next level by giving you the opportunity to illustrate new skills in the moment and model a new pattern of responding for parents.

Interventions with Children and Adolescents

Emotions have an important physiological component and teaching youth strategies for calming the physiological effects of emotions is a critical emotion regulation strategy. These strategies can be used at any level of emotional arousal, including highly dysregulated states, which makes them essential tools for undercontrolled youth. Overcontrolled youth also benefit from learning these strategies as it increases their self-efficacy in coping with emotions and will likely increase their willingness to participate in emotional exposures.

For each of these strategies, introduce the technique (you can use the script provided), practice the skill in session with the child, provide corrective feedback, repeat your practice, and troubleshoot how the child can remember to practice at home and to use the skill in times of stress. Don't forget that parents should be learning these same skills!

Children do not need to know any basics about emotions in order to benefit from these strategies. If you can get them to practice emotion regulation techniques designed to reduce physiological arousal, this will be effective whether they understand emotions or not. You can immediately introduce and practice these skills with a child who, for example, presents in a highly dysregulated state and is unlikely to be able to participate in other interventions. However, children may learn *more* from these strategies if they know (1) how to identify and label their emotions, (2) that emotions have a physiological component, and (3) that emotions can be different intensities (see the Facts about Feelings intervention). If the child understands that emotions can have different intensities, have the child rate his or her emotion before and after each practice.

Off to the Races (overcontrol and undercontrol)

Ages: 4–12 years.

Module: Basic Behavioral Tasks.

Purpose: Teach children to regulate the physiological component of emotions.

Rationale: Targeting physiological sensations is an effective strategy for regulating emotions and one way to do this is to slow down one's breathing.

Materials: Paper boat and instructions for folding a paper boat (HQ Card 5.8, Building a Boat, p. 112).

Expected time needed: 5 minutes (plus 5 minutes preparation).

This *Express* strategy is easy to learn, fun, and effective, which means that youth quickly build self-efficacy in using these skills. Children who struggle with emotion dysregulation often believe it will be very difficult or even impossible for them to change how they feel, so it is essential for them to have successful experiences with emotion regulation skills early on. Physiological arousal is closely tied to emotional intensity. It is very hard to feel calm when one's breathing is rapid. Off to the Races is an engaging way to get children to practice calming their bodies by taking long, slow breaths.

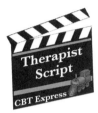

What the Therapist Can Say

"Have you ever noticed that when we get upset we start breathing really fast? I know when I'm [nervous/scared/angry] I sometimes start to go [*demonstrates rapid, shallow breathing*]. When we breathe in fast and shallow like that, it grows our emotion and makes it hard to calm down. A really good way to calm our emotions is to slow down our breathing, and we're going to practice one way to do that right now. We are going to have a paper boat race, right here on this table! Here's your boat and I've got mine. I'm going to tell you a trick—if you take a nice deep breath and then blow all the air out really slow and long like this [*demonstrates*], your boat will float farther across the table-lake! Let's give it a try."

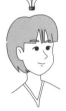

What the Therapist Can Do

Depending on the age/interest of the child and the amount of time you have, you can either fold paper boats together or have them prepared ahead of time. It only takes a few minutes to fold a couple of paper boats, so you can explain deep breathing while folding boats together with a child. Make sure to give a printout of the paper boat folding instructions to the family to take home. Encourage parents to play Off to the Races with their child.

4–5–6 (overcontrol and undercontrol)

Ages: 13 years and older.

Module: Basic Behavioral Tasks.

Purpose: Teach teens to regulate the physiological component of emotions.

Rationale: Targeting physiological sensations is an effective strategy for regulating emotions and one way to do this is to slow down one's breathing.

Materials: None.

Expected time needed: 5 minutes.

Similar to Off to the Races for younger children, 4–5–6 is a quick and engaging way for teens to build self-efficacy in reducing physiological arousal. Teens are just as likely as younger children to be skeptical that they have the power to change their emotions, so helping them practice effective strategies for calming their bodies will help get buy-in that these strategies really do work!

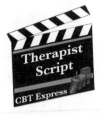

What the Therapist Can Say

"I bet it seems silly to practice breathing—you already do it all the time! But here's the thing, often when we get upset, our breathing starts to get like this [*demonstrates fast, shallow breaths*]. Every time we breathe in, we are amping up that emotion and when we breathe out, we turn the volume down. So it makes sense if our brain thinks we're in danger, we're gonna take in a lot of oxygen to get ourselves ready to get away. But if we want to calm down, we want to do the opposite—start slowing down our breaths and making the exhale longer than the inhale. That tells our brain to turn down the emotion volume and helps us relax. One way to remember this is to think 4–5–6. First, we'll breathe in for a count of 4, hold our breath for 5, and then exhale for 6. Let's do it together. Breathe in . . . 2 . . . 3 . . . 4 . . . Hold . . . 2 . . . 3 . . . 4 . . . 5 . . . Breathe out . . . 2 . . . 3 . . . 4 . . . 5 . . . 6 . . . [*repeat three times*]."

Angry Sponge/Anxious Sponge (overcontrol and undercontrol)

Ages: 4–12 years old.

Module: Basic Behavioral Tasks.

Purpose: Teach children to regulate the physiological component of emotions.

Rationale: Targeting physiological sensations is an effective strategy for regulating emotions and one way to do this is to relax muscles.

Expected time needed: 5 minutes each.

Materials: Sponge and water.

This intervention is an interactive way to help children practice relaxing their bodies. Based on progressive muscle relaxation, a technique that has been used for decades (Carlson & Holye, 1993), Angry Sponge/Anxious Sponge takes what can be a complex procedure for adults and simplifies it into a fun activity that even young children can understand. Using the image of a sponge absorbing and releasing water, children will vividly remember this intervention. Children can even be given a small sponge to keep in a place where they often become dysregulated—on their desk at home, in their backpack at school—as a reminder to practice this skill.

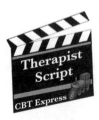

What the Therapist Can Say

"Sometimes we can soak up anger all through the day until it builds up and up and up. It's sort of like if I take a sponge and put it under some running water [*run water, soak sponge*], it gets filled up with water. Your body is like an angry sponge and the way to get the anger out is to SQUEEZE [*demonstrate squeezing sponge*]. Let's try it with our bodies this time and get all the angries out! Standing [*sitting/lying down*] right here, I want you to think about all those things making you angry and then when I say "Squeeze," you're going to squeeze all your muscles to get those angry feelings out! Ready? 1–2–3–SQUEEZE! Squeeze your muscles really tight! OK, relax. Usually one squeeze isn't enough, let's squeeze some more. 1–2–3–SQUEEEEEEEEZE! And relax. Ooooh, I could see a lot of angries coming out that time. Let's do it again! 1–2–3–SQUEEZE! And relax. Nice one!"

What the Therapist Can Do

This activity can be adapted to focus on the emotion that is most difficult for the particular child. For example, a child who gets tense due to feeling anxious can squeeze the worries out of her Anxious Sponge. It's OK not to demonstrate with an actual sponge if you don't have the materials available, but make sure you practice with the child. Have parents practice as well so that they can model and reinforce the use of this technique at home. Don't just tell the child what to do. Show her how to tense all her muscles up by scrunching up her face, making tight fists, and tightening her stomach, arms, and legs.

The following *Express* interventions are designed to help children shift their focus. Attentional control is one of the first emotion regulation strategies children display (Gross, 1998). From a young age, babies can be seen averting their gaze when emotionally distressed, and young children often cover their eyes when scared (Gross, 1998). Distraction techniques can be used by undercontrolled children when attending to an emotionally salient stimulus is leading to emotion dysregulation. When they shift their focus to a neutral or pleasant stimuli for a period of time, their emotional arousal can decrease, allowing them to respond more adaptively to the emotion. Note that these strategies are not recommended for overcontrolled youth, who tend to be emotionally avoidant and may overuse distraction techniques.

Alphabetical Animals (undercontrol)

Ages: 6 years and older.

Module: Basic Behavioral Tasks.

Purpose: Teach children and teens to use distraction to regulate emotions.

Rationale: Undercontrolled youth may become "triggered" by an emotionally salient stimulus and continue to focus on it while they become dysregulated. Learning to shift one's focus to a neutral or positive stimulus can help undercontrolled youth decrease emotional arousal quickly.

Materials: None.

Expected time needed: 5 minutes.

Alphabetical Animals teaches children and teens how to shift their focus when emotions are overwhelming. When they pick a neutral or even positive category like animals, chances are that after just a few minutes of playing this game, their emotions will come down at least a little. The goal of these shifting focus activities is exactly that—it teaches children how to take enough of an emotional break so that they can jump back in and approach the problem with a calmer mind.

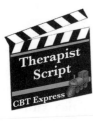

What the Therapist Can Say

"Sometimes when emotions are strong, we need a break, and it helps to focus on something different for a few minutes. Emotions really grab our attention and this makes us focus more on whatever it is that set off the emotion. For example, if someone teases me, I would feel sad, and I might spend a lot of time thinking about what that person said. I might even start thinking about other mean things people have said, and that's going to keep me feeling really sad. It might help me figure out what to do next if I first take a break from thinking about teasing, but it's really hard to just stop thinking about something. Let's try an experiment. If I say: don't think about a green dog! What did you think about? I bet you thought of a green dog! It's really hard to just not think about something, even if we really want to. It works better to get some different thoughts in your mind or to do something different; this can be a good way to distract yourself for a little bit if emotions are really strong.

"Let's try one way together: Name an animal for each letter of the alphabet. You can choose a different category than animals if you want, like Disney characters, football teams, or movies. Remember, you don't get graded, so it's OK if you get stuck. You can skip a letter, change categories, or make up something new!"

Here's an example of playing alphabetical animals with 7-year-old Kimiko, who was sobbing because she was afraid of getting an injection.

THERAPIST: Kimiko, do you like animals?

KIMIKO: (*sobbing*) I don't want to get a shot!

THERAPIST: I know. Let's play a game—we're going to name animals for each letter of the alphabet. What's an animal that starts with *A*?

KIMIKO: (*gasping*) I . . . don't . . . know.

THERAPIST: Hmm . . . how about . . . alligator! OK! How about *B*?

KIMIKO: (*Sniffles.*) . . . bear?

THERAPIST: Oh, that's a great one! I like bears. I can see a *C* animal on your shirt!

KIMIKO: (*Looks down.*) Cat.

THERAPIST: Yep! OK, *D* . . . dinosaur!

KIMIKO: That doesn't count. They're not alive.

THERAPIST: Oh, I guess you're right. What *D* animal can you think of?

KIMIKO: *Dog!*

THERAPIST: You know a lot of animals! What's next?

KIMIKO: *E. Elephant!* Now you do *F*.

Face Your Feelings (overcontrol and undercontrol)

Ages: 4 years and older.

Module: Behavioral Experiments and Exposures.

Purpose: Decreasing avoidance of emotions and modifying beliefs about emotions by increasing youths' ability to tolerate experiencing and expressing emotions.

Rationale: As with targeting fears in other areas, exposures designed to decrease avoidance and challenge maladaptive predictions help increase youths' ability to tolerate emotional situations, increase their self-efficacy with respect to emotional expression, and modify maladaptive beliefs.

Materials: None.

Expected time needed: 15 minutes.

Often, overcontrolled children have fears about expressing emotions. They might hold catastrophic beliefs about what will occur if they experience and express emotions (e.g., "It will never end"; "I won't be able to handle it"; "Everyone will think I'm weak and stupid") and as a result, they avoid emotionally salient experiences. Just as graduated exposure is critical to the treatment of any other fear, overcontrolled children benefit from graduated exposure to emotion.

Undercontrolled youth may also end up avoiding emotions, but in different ways. They may have such an intense emotional response to stimuli that it is difficult for them to tolerate the emotion without responding impulsively. They may quickly resort to destructive emotion regulation strategies—like an angry child who throws a chair, then feels guilty and cries until he's worn out and falls asleep. This pattern interrupts the natural course of the initial emotion. The anger, if tolerated, will eventually decrease and dissipate. The impulsive action (throwing the chair) and the secondary emotion (guilt) essentially lead to the child avoiding the experience of anger. Emotion exposures for undercontrolled children allow the child to experience that the feeling can be tolerated without responding impulsively and that emotions will decrease naturally with time.

For both overcontrolled and undercontrolled youth, emotion exposure involves creating a fear hierarchy beginning with mildly feared emotions or emotional situations and continuing to the most feared emotional event. If you are new to exposure as an intervention, see Chapter 6 for further details on implementing exposure effectively.

It is essential that children know some basics about emotions in order to benefit from exposure techniques. Start with the *Express* intervention Facts about Feelings to be sure the child has a solid understanding of these important aspects of emotion. Then the child will be ready for Face Your Feelings.

The general steps for doing an emotion exposure are the same, but each specific exposure must be tailored to the child. See the steps below, followed by examples of exposures to various types of emotions.

1. Orient the child to the exposure.
2. Conduct the exposure.
3. Draw the child's attention to the experience and expression of emotion.
4. Rate emotional intensity.
5. Highlight lessons learned.

Exposures to Fear

For children who avoid fear-inducing situations, the strategies for designing exposures are identical to those you would use for anxiety disorders. See Chapter 6 for more details on these critical interventions. Consider activities such as watching portions of a scary movie, discussing a frightening experience, or imagining a feared scenario.

Exposures to Joy

Some overcontrolled children will even avoid expressing feelings of happiness and joy. These exposures are particularly fun to do! Consider activities such as watching funny animal videos online, looking through photos on the child's phone, describing a pleasant memory, reading a joke book, or watching a comedian or portions of a funny movie or TV show.

Exposures to Anger

Many overcontrolled children avoid experiencing or expressing anger. For some, even seeing others express anger is highly uncomfortable. Exposures may begin with watching a scene from a TV show or movie that involves someone being angry. Try to pick a scene depicting a character who resembles the child you are working with in age and gender. Other activities to consider include acting out an angry role play, making angry faces, and discussing a situation that made the child angry.

Exposures to Sadness

Overcontrolled children may avoid experiencing and especially expressing sadness; they often avoid crying, particularly in front of others. Watching sad movies and TV, listening to sad music (consider the background music of sad scenes in movies or songs a teen associates with a sad memory), viewing images of people crying, making sad faces, putting eye drops in to mimic the sensation of crying, and acting out a sad role play are all activities that can be used for sadness exposures.

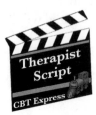

What the Therapist Can Say

"Remember when you learned to ride a bike [play the piano, throw a football]? I bet the first time you tried, it was pretty hard. It might have been scary or difficult, and you may not have been able to do it quite right. Over time, with practice, I bet you got better and better until now it's easy to do and you're much better at it than you were when you started. Facing our feelings takes practice too—it can be pretty scary and hard at first, but if we practice, it gets easier and more comfortable. If in the very beginning when you were learning to ride a bike, you stopped at the first sign of difficulty, you wouldn't be able to do it at all today! When we face our feelings, it works the same way. If we stop when it gets hard, we don't get the chance to see that it actually gets easier and we get better at it the more we practice.

"A lot of kids have trouble facing their feelings. Sometimes they might do things to try to avoid facing feelings, like running away, hiding their face, closing their eyes, or turning away. What are the ways you stop facing feelings? Together we'll be on the lookout for those signs of avoiding—as soon as we notice them, we'll remind ourselves to face our feelings by walking back, uncovering our faces, opening our eyes wide, and looking our feelings right on.

"We're going to practice facing joy [fear/anger/sadness] together. The way we do that is we do something together that makes us feel joyful [scared/angry/sad]. When we do, I'll ask you where you feel the joy [fear/anger/sadness] in your body, and I want you to try your best to describe it. Don't worry if it's hard at first—remember, it'll get easier with practice. We are also going to rate how strong our feelings of joy [fear/anger/sadness] are from 0–10. At the end, we'll decide what we learned. Are you ready to face joy [fear/anger/sadness] with me?"

What the Therapist Can Do

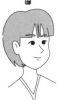

Therapists should work with the child on feeling identification. Begin by discussing, thinking about, reading about, or watching others expressing emotions. Picture books, videos, and movie clips can be excellent tools.

Next, collaborate with families to evoke past emotional experiences that are rated at varying intensities on the child's emotion scale. Have the child describe feeling the target emotion at a 2, 5, and 10. Encourage the child to include as much detail as she can recall; what did she feel, think, hear, see, taste, touch, and smell? Write down her descriptions and read them aloud if repeated exposure is needed at this step.

You will want to elicit emotions when possible and appropriate. After prepping the child for emotional exposure, including the rationale and process, be attuned to changes in emotion and ask the child to describe and experience that emotion intensely. Bring the child's attention to his feelings, thoughts, body sensations, and action urges. Notice efforts to avoid emotions by changing the topic, looking away, hiding his face, and so forth. Have the child repeatedly rate emotional intensity. You can do this using numbers (e.g., 0–10) or using the arm as a lever, with the elbow bent and hand pointing straight up as maximum intensity and elbow bent with hand pointing straight forward as minimum intensity. The child can raise and lower his arm throughout the exposure to indicate emotional distress. It is critical for the child to learn that he can tolerate remaining at a high level of emotional intensity. Rating emotional intensity allows the child to observe that emotions do not last forever and intensity will change over time.

Finally, practice appropriate emotion regulation in session while the child is emotionally aroused. Do not rush to this stage, as learning that one can handle emotional intensity without escaping or suppressing emotional expression is critical for overcontrolled youth. If the child agrees to participate in an emotional exposure for 5 minutes, when the time is up, this would be a great time to practice with the child Off to the Races or 4–5–6 skills described previously. This will allow the child to end the emotional exposure through adaptive emotion regulation, which builds self-efficacy and increases willingness to continue to participate in exposures.

If you're thinking this sounds like a lot to do in an *Express* intervention, you're right! The key part is to get the child and family up and running in your brief intervention, so that they are able to continue these kinds of exposures on their own. Think of exposure as a change in lifestyle, not a one-off treatment. If you were supporting a family in eating healthier, you might provide the rationale and help them develop a meal plan in person, but the day-to-day choices about healthier eating need to occur over and over again every day. Exposure works the same way. For example, you might create a hierarchy and do one exposure in a 10-minute meeting with the family, then assign homework to repeat that exposure each day until it's easy, then move up the exposure hierarchy.

Conclusion

Emotion dysregulation can be a challenging presenting concern. Keeping the interactions with families focused and utilizing *Express* interventions can help increase skills in regulation and prevent future worsening of symptoms. The following tips will help you keep interventions with families on the *Express* track and not get derailed by emotion dysregulation.

1. Practice! Don't just teach the skill, have the child and parent practice the techniques in session.
2. Give corrective feedback and practice again.
3. Don't forget to troubleshoot how the child and parent can remember to use these skills at home.
4. Remember that parents need to learn each emotion regulation skill the child learns. This is essential because parents are the ones who can coach children through adaptive emotion regulation between sessions. In addition, parents of emotionally dysregulated children are likely to struggle with emotion regulation themselves. By learning emotion regulation techniques, they can reduce their own emotional dysregulation (which allows them to parent more effectively) and model appropriate emotion regulation for the child.

Facts about Feelings

Feelings are important and can help us out.	Describe a time when you felt SAD, SCARED, or ANGRY and it was helpful. How did the feeling help you?
Feelings aren't always accurate.	Describe a time when you felt SAD, SCARED, or ANGRY and it was not accurate. This could be something you were afraid of that was not dangerous or a time when you felt angry because of something you thought happened but really did not.
Feelings have different components.	Pick a situation where you felt a strong feeling and complete the following sections. What was the situation (e.g., starting a new job)? _____ _____ Name the feeling (e.g., anxiety). _____
Feelings have different intensities. Feelings don't last forever.	How strong was the feeling from 0–10? _____ What thoughts did you have (e.g., "I won't be able to handle it")? _____ _____ What sensations did you feel in your body (e.g., sweaty, heart racing)? _____ What actions did you take (e.g., arrived early)? _____ _____ When did the feeling change (e.g., 20 minutes, the next day)? _____ _____

Is This Valid?: Parental Validation Practice

Pick the most validating response.

1. I'm never going to finish this project. I keep screwing it up! My teacher is going to be so mad at me.
   a. This is why I told you to start a month ago! You're always leaving things to the last minute.
   b. You'll finish. You're so creative and smart. I just know your teacher is going to love it—she always does!
   c. You seem really stressed. I bet it's hard to finish when you're overwhelmed and worried about the outcome.

2. I can't believe you won't let me go to the party! Everyone is going to be there and I'll just be the loser whose parents are strict. You are literally ruining my life.
   a. I know you are very disappointed by our decision. I can understand that being with your friends is really important to you.
   b. You are so ungrateful! I don't care that everyone else is going—as long as you live in my house, you follow my rules.
   c. Come on, it's just one party. No one will even remember if you're there or not.

3. [Tearful] Betty said she hates me and will never be my friend again.
   a. I'm sure Betty doesn't hate you! She is your best friend and you guys will get over it by tomorrow, like you always do.
   b. You must feel really sad that she said that. I know how much you care about her as a friend.
   c. Calm down, she doesn't mean it. You need to stop getting so upset over little things.

4. ARGH! I hate math homework! I'm never going to get it—I'm just too dumb.
   a. You're not dumb! There are so many things you're good at—you just need to work harder instead of giving up.
   b. Quit complaining and just focus on your work. I don't want to spend three hours on one assignment like we did last night.
   c. I understand you're feeling frustrated—it's really hard sticking with something that's difficult.

5. Nooooooo, I can't go in the pool!
   a. I don't want to hear any more of this whining—just do it.
   b. Okay okay, you don't have to.
   c. It's pretty scary doing something new for the first time, isn't it?

No "Buts" Allowed!

When you want to validate your child, a good rule of thumb is to avoid the word "but." That does not mean you have to agree with what your child is doing or wants to do; it just means paying attention to the language you use. It might sound funny at first AND you can get the hang of it with practice (see what I did there?). Turn these invalidating "buts" into "but"-free validations.

Example: I get that you want to hang out with your friends, BUT it is just too late to get home at midnight. Your curfew is 10:00 P.M.

"But"-free: I get that you want to hang out with your friends AND I'm still not comfortable with you getting home at midnight. Your curfew is 10:00 P.M.

I can tell you're really upset, BUT we are going to be late for school!
"But"-free:

It makes sense to be angry when someone does that, BUT you need to get over it so you can finish your project.
"But"-free:

I know you're scared of going on stage, BUT you've practiced so hard. You're going to do great.
"But"-free:"

You seem really hurt by what Priya said, BUT I'm sure she didn't mean it.
"But"-free:

I understand you're feeling sad, BUT you still need to do your chores.
"But"-free:

Amp Up Expression

This handout will help you increase adaptive emotional expression in your child.

First, identify one to three behaviors you want to increase. These are ways you would like your child to express his or her emotions more frequently. For example, for an overcontrolled child, you may want to increase labeling emotions and expressing sadness, while for an undercontrolled child, expressing anger calmly may be the goal.

Next, come up with reinforcers you can use for each behavior. See the example below and then fill in a few ways you can "amp up expression" with your child.

	Example: Label emotions	Target behavior:	Target behavior:	Target behavior:
Validate	"It makes sense that you're feeling sad."			
Praise	"I really appreciate you telling me how you feel."			
Give attention	Hug			

Catch Them Using Skills

This handout will help you increase adaptive emotional regulation in your child.

First, identify one to three regulation strategies you want your child to use more frequently. For example, your child might be learning deep breathing, relaxation, and distraction.

Next, come up with reinforcers you can use for each behavior.

	Example: Deep breathing	Target behavior:	Target behavior:	Target behavior:
Praise	"Wow, you are getting really good at that deep breathing!"			
Give attention	High-5			
Reward	Trip to the park (20 points)			

Reward Chart: Sample

If you decide to use rewards to increase a specific behavior, it is important to have a way to keep track of points a child earns toward those rewards. Points should be given immediately following the behavior, while rewards might be worth many points and be earned only after a child has engaged in the behavior many times. Use the handy chart and reward menu below as a guide. First you'll see an example that Priya's parents used and then there's a blank copy for you.

	Monday	Tuesday	Wednesday	Thursday	Friday	Saturday	Sunday
Target behavior: Deep breathing	★			★	★		
Target behavior: Drawing		★			★		
Target behavior: Playing with Toto		★		★		★	★
Total Points	1	2	0	2	2	1	1
						Week Total	9

Priya_____'s Reward Menu	
Reward	**Points**
20 minutes of screen time	5 points
Trip to the park with Toto	10 points
Movie night	15 points
Sleepover	20 points

Reward Chart

	Monday	Tuesday	Wednesday	Thursday	Friday	Saturday	Sunday
Target behavior:							
Target behavior:							
Target behavior:							
Total Points							
					Week Total		

_____'s Reward Menu	
Reward	**Points**

Don't Throw Fuel on the Fire

Parents of undercontrolled children are often unintentionally reinforcing maladaptive behavior—sort of like throwing fuel on the fire. In order to change this pattern parents need to catch this unintentional reinforcement (the fuel) and increase reinforcement of adaptive behavior.

The Old Cycle

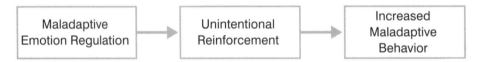

The Fire: Maladaptive emotion regulation	The Fuel: Unintentional reinforcement	Even Bigger Fire: Increased maladaptive behavior
Suresh throws a tantrum at the grocery store because he wants a toy car.	Suresh's father buys the toy and says, "Next time you better behave or you're not getting anything."	More tantrums
Celia hits her sister Grace because Grace took Celia's puzzle.	Celia's mother lectures Celia for 30 minutes about not hitting her sister.	More hitting
Jorge cuts his leg after getting dumped by his girlfriend.	Jorge's mother spends an hour bandaging Jorge's leg while crying, telling Jorge how much she loves him, and asking him to never do this again.	More cutting

(continued)

Don't Throw Fuel on the Fire (page 2 of 2)

Break the Cycle

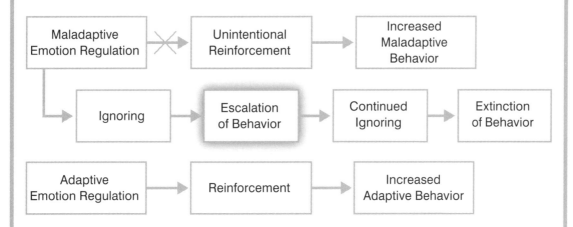

To break the cycle, parents need to put out small fires by IGNORING, while fueling adaptive emotion regulation. Ignoring a behavior that you were previously reinforcing with attention will lead to extinction, as long as you tolerate and don't reinforce the inevitable extinction burst!

Here is an example of how Suresh's family was able to break the cycle.

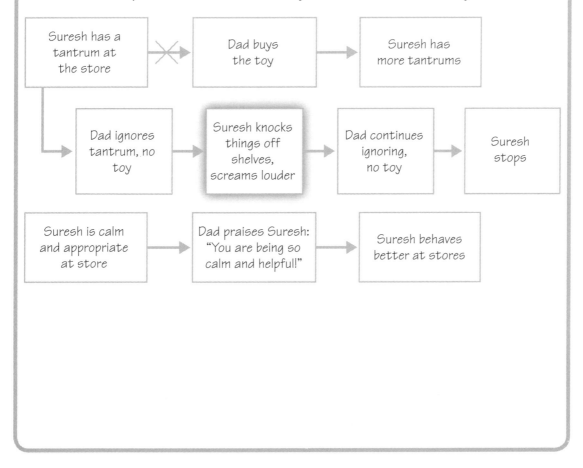

Building a Boat

Fears and Worries

"She hates trying new things."

"Everything worries him—if it is raining, he worries about tornadoes; if it is sunny, he worries about skin cancer."

"If his schedule get changed he just melts down."

"She gets so worked up about shots and just cries and says she can't."

Whether it is a fear of an imminent shot during a well-child check or anxiety about attending school, fears and worries are often identified as a concern by families when they seek help in primary care settings, mental health clinics, therapists' offices, or in school counselors' offices. Symptoms can range from annoyance to debilitating panic. Anxiety is one of the most frequent reasons children are referred for mental health services, and can also arise as a problem in other health care settings. Anxiety symptoms can benefit from brief, in vivo interventions that require little introduction for families and thus are ideal for quick and effective evidence-based interventions in schools, primary care settings, or mental health treatment settings in the context of other care, as well as when a full "traditional" therapy hour cannot be devoted to one intervention.

Brief Statement Regarding Evidence-Based Treatments

CBT is the evidence-based treatment approach for a variety of anxiety disorders and symptoms. Behavioral interventions provide youth with new coping skills and ways to tolerate distress while cognitive interventions help children learn how to spot thinking errors and generate more balanced thoughts (Seligman & Ollendick, 2011; Weersing, Rozenman, Maher-Bridge, & Campo, 2012). Exposures are the most vital component in the treatment of childhood anxiety disorders, as they cement learning and provide youth with the opportunity to master their fears (Tiwari, Kendall, Hoff, Harrison & Fizur, 2013).

Considerations such as age, gender, race, ethnicity, and severity of symptom presentation do not moderate outcomes (Kendall & Peterman, 2015; Walkup et al., 2008). Using CBT to treat symptoms of anxiety yields reductions in symptom severity, improvements in global functioning, enhancements in social functioning, and reductions in sleep disturbances (Higa-McMillan, Francis, Rith-Najarian, & Chorpita, 2016; Pereira et al., 2016; Peterman et al., 2016; Walkup et al., 2008). A recent comprehensive review of anxiety studies noted that children who participated in CBT conditions were three to seven times more likely to show significant improvements in anxiety symptoms (Bennett et al., 2016).

Innovative approaches seek to increase the dissemination of CBT for anxious youth. CBT can be effectively supplemented and augmented using a variety of computer-based programs or mobile device applications (Kendall & Peterman, 2015; Reyes-Portillo et al., 2014). Hundreds of applications currently exist that facilitate the generalization of behavioral and cognitive tools (Berry & Lai, 2014; Elkins, McHugh, Santucci, & Barlow, 2011). Furthermore, research shows that brief packages of CBT are just as effective as more extensive protocols, as long as active learning is emphasized throughout treatment (Crawley et al., 2013). In other words, the *Express* interventions in this chapter present an excellent opportunity for clinicians to provide the exact care that young patients need to win the battle against their fears and worries.

Presenting Concerns and Symptoms

Anxiety disorders and symptoms are highly treatable, but many children's symptoms go unrecognized and therefore untreated. When a child presents with anxiety symptoms in any setting, it is an opportunity to quickly demonstrate for the child and family how effective CBT can be. A therapist's ability to immediately describe the powerful nature of CBT may convince otherwise reluctant families to engage in treatment. To quickly show the benefits of CBT, therapists must efficiently assess the level of anxiety, the child's understanding of his symptoms, and his willingness and ability to initially engage in interventions. However, a child's lack of ability to engage in interventions during the interaction does not mean the opportunity is lost. The child can learn by watching you model techniques, and parents can develop skills and gain knowledge about interventions they can apply later at home. Keep in mind that anxiety symptoms may manifest in a variety of ways, including anxious or worried affect, vocalization of fears, difficulty transitioning, somatic symptoms, sleep disturbance, tantrums/behavioral issues, and compulsive behaviors. Further, because of the overlap of anxiety symptoms among anxiety diagnoses, the interventions can each be modified and applied to most anxiety-related presenting concerns or diagnoses.

Interventions

Children with lots of worries, such as those with generalized anxiety disorder (GAD), carry around a great burden of anxiety. Whatever seems to be going on, their thoughts go to the worst scenarios or catastrophic outcomes, and they experience feelings of helplessness.

For some families, GAD poses more challenges than other types of anxiety disorders because the target of the worries continuously shifts. These families often find themselves in a cycle of providing reassurance for the various concerns expressed by the child, and the child takes on more and more burdens, seeing the world as a dangerous, unpredictable place. Although parents intend to help the child by providing reassurance, this backfires by reinforcing the worrying pattern and holds the symptoms in place. Many of the strategies in this chapter can easily be applied to the specific fear or worry impacting a patient with GAD at any one time, but to address the ongoing symptoms and compounding impact of these fears on children, the Don't Sink the Boat intervention can be effective in illustrating the cycle of worrying and reassurance.

Don't Sink the Boat

Ages: 7 years and older and parents.

Module: Psychoeducation.

Purpose: Provide family with information on the cycle of anxiety and the unintended consequences of providing reassurance to the child.

Rationale: Families often don't realize that the reassurance they are providing is actually reinforcing the anxiety symptoms, and that to reduce the anxiety they need to stop this cycle.

Materials: HQ Card 6.1, Don't Sink the Boat (p. 130), or paper and a writing utensil (optional: toy boat).

Expected time needed: 10–15 minutes.

Worries burden children, and it is painful for parents to watch them continuously dragged down by worry. Don't Sink the Boat is a strategy for reminding children and their families not to let the worries pile up like rocks in a boat and weigh them down. The strategy reminds them to take control of their thoughts and toss the unhelpful worries overboard to prevent the boat from sinking. Sometimes parents get into the pattern of bailing out the water to "rescue" the child, but when children keep adding more rocks into the boat, the boat just takes on more water. Rather, parents need to learn how to help their children get rid of the rocks, which will eventually alleviate the underlying problem.

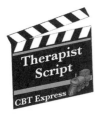

What the Therapist Can Say

"Sounds like you feel worried a lot of the time about lots of different things. Those worries are really weighing you down. If you think about sitting in a small boat and see each of your worries as a large rock being added to the boat, what do you think happens as you add more and more worries? That's right, the boat gets heavier and heavier and starts to take on water. And, you start to feel more anxious and panicked. You might ask your parents for reassurance, which is like scooping out a little water—it helps a little but only for a brief time. What we really need to do is figure out how to get the rocks out so you don't sink the boat. Are you ready to throw some of those worries overboard?"

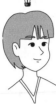

What the Therapist Can Do

The therapist can use a toy boat to illustrate this concept. Families are instructed to write worries on small pieces of paper that they ball up like rocks. The worries are put into the boat. Children then practice throwing the worries overboard while parents avoid providing reassurance. Families can then use this metaphor as a short cut for talking about worries at home. If a child is seeking reassurance regarding a particular worry, the parents can state, "Sounds like another rock in your boat—throw it overboard!" HQ Card 6.1 provides drawings of rocks to prompt children to identify specific worries to use during this *Express* intervention.

Over the River and through the Woods

Ages: 7 years and older; parents of children of all ages.

Module: Psychoeducation.

Purpose: Increase families' understanding of the connection between thoughts and feelings.

Rationale: If families understand how thoughts and feelings are connected, they may be more likely to implement cognitive modification strategies with the understanding that the interventions will lead to relief of anxiety symptoms.

Materials: HQ Card 6.2, Over the River and through the Woods (p. 131), and a writing utensil.

Expected time needed: 5 minutes.

Helping families understand the connection between thoughts and feelings is a key part of the role of a therapist working with anxious children. When families understand the connection, they better understand the purpose of the interventions being introduced, and with increased understanding they may be more likely to follow through with the use of the strategies and further treatment, if needed. "Over the River and through the Woods" is a popular song based on a poem first published in 1844 by Lydia Maria Child, and since it is familiar to many families it may be easier for them to remember this strategy by thinking of the song. This intervention helps families remember how thoughts and feelings are connected, and how modifying thoughts can lead to changes in feelings. The introductory script below can be used to quickly illustrate the connection for families. Therapists can modify it to speak more directly to parents if the patient is younger, or to talk directly to the child or teen, depending on the setting and cognitive development of the child.

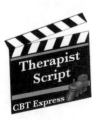

What the Therapist Can Say

"You have shared several symptoms of anxiety that occur most days. The feelings you (or your child) are describing, including nervousness, anxiety, and worry, are connected to the thoughts you are having—for example, when you say to yourself [*insert thought the child/family shared if possible*], 'What if I fail the exam?,' what happens to your anxious and worried feelings? That's right, they get stronger. And the more thoughts you have like that the stronger and stronger the feelings get and the harder it is to switch to another path. Think of your thoughts like a path in the woods that starts off overgrown. The more you go down the same path, the more your brain remembers it. It becomes a clearer path, and you start to take that path automatically. The song 'Over the River and through the Woods' can remind you of this pattern. What is the next line in the song? That's right—'to Grandmother's house we go.' In the song, they know the path to Grandmother's house and take it automatically because they have likely been there before. Your worry path is similar. You have taken the path so many times that your thoughts automatically go down that well-worn path, which leads to more worry feelings. We want to create a new path so that the worry feelings lessen. How does that sound?"

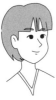

What the Therapist Can Do

Therapists can use HQ Card 6.2 to demonstrate the paths and have the child trace various paths with a pencil or crayon, illustrating how much darker and more pronounced the path becomes with repetition. It can also be helpful for therapists to explain this *CBT Express* intervention to parents and/or children by describing what happens when you take a stick and draw a line in the sand. The more you trace that same line, the more pronounced the line in the sand becomes and the harder it is to push the stick off the grooved path to create a new path. Therapists can then work with families to identify what the new path might be and how to practice those adaptive, modified thoughts throughout the week in order to strengthen that path.

My Worry Tree

Ages: 10 years and older and parents.

Module: Psychoeducation.

Purpose: Teach families about how thoughts stem from beliefs children have about themselves, others and the world.

Rationale: Understanding where their thoughts are coming from can help children and teens work to challenge the beliefs that are triggering maladaptive and inaccurate thoughts.

Materials: HQ Cards 6.3a and 6.3b, My Worry Tree, sample and blank cards (pp. 132–134), and a writing utensil; scissors; tape.

Expected time needed: 15 minutes.

My Worry Tree provides families with a visual representation of the child's growing worries. Therapists can use HQ Cards 6.3a and 6.3b to illustrate how beliefs (the trunk) can lead to more specific fears (branches) and automatic thoughts (leaves). The branches or fears keep growing more leaves, just like inaccurate beliefs lead to distorted thoughts. This *Express* exercise involves coaching children to let the worry leaves fall off the tree like the leaves in autumn, and grow new leaves by challenging and changing their beliefs.

For example, Ty was experiencing social anxiety. He viewed the world as a dangerous place, and he ignored his ability to cope with social situations when he was in different settings, like school, soccer practice, or sleepovers. My Worry Tree is introduced with a script like the one below and then completed with the child in the *Express* session. Paper leaves are cut out and labeled with fear-based automatic thoughts and then turned over and replaced with more balanced and coping thoughts.

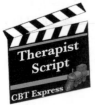

What the Therapist Can Say

"It seems your worries are tricking you into believing the world is a dangerous place and making you think you can't cope with the situations in your life. This belief is like the trunk of this tree. Viewing the world this way leads to fears in certain situations, which are like these branches. You have fears about school, soccer, and sleepovers. Then those fears lead to thoughts that pop into your head when you think about or encounter those situations. Those thoughts are like the leaves on this tree. Some of the thoughts you shared are 'The other kids will laugh at me,' 'I will get hurt and look stupid in front of the team,' and 'The other kids will think I am annoying.' Let's write those down on the leaves on this worksheet."

What the Therapist Can Do

The therapist then works with the child to write down the beliefs and thoughts. The leaves that contain the maladaptive thoughts are discussed using Socratic questioning and guided discovery techniques. Self-instruction prompts can also be used to help youth identify new thoughts and then write those modified thoughts on the other side of the leaves (e.g., "Just because _____ doesn't mean _____"). Families can be taught to continue to work on these modifications, and then cross out the beliefs on the trunk and replace them with new beliefs as the child progresses.

De-Ice Your Fears

Ages: 7 years and older.

Module: Cognitive Restructuring.

Purpose: De-ice (change) thoughts through self-instruction and cognitive modification to reduce anxiety and promote coping and problem solving.

Rationale: Modifying maladaptive and inaccurate thoughts can increase children's ability to engage in feared activities, including exposures, and reduce the intensity of the anxious feelings.

Materials: HQ Cards 6.4a and 6.4b, De-Ice Your Fears, sample and blank cards (pp. 135–136), and a writing utensil.

Expected time needed: 15 minutes.

The intensity of fears, especially phobias, can sometimes surprise parents and providers. Anxiety can start subtly and through inadvertent reinforcement grow to the point where it impacts the functioning not only of the child but the other family members as well. Phobias vary regarding the specific object or situation that is feared, but the approach for intervention is similar regardless. In addition to the other *Express* exposure interventions below (e.g.,

Exposure, Exposure, Exposure and Kick Up the Dirt), therapists can use cognitive restructuring and self-talk to modify maladaptive and inaccurate thoughts. These techniques will help modify erroneous or unhelpful thoughts and can increase the child's willingness and motivation to engage in exposure work. The *Express* intervention De-Ice Your Fears will help you do so quickly and effectively.

Fears can be debilitating, and can feel like they are freezing a person, leaving him or her unable to cope, problem solve, or think rationally. De-Ice Your Fears is a quick, easy-to-remember strategy designed to help children with anxiety regain control and manage their fear. It can be tailored to younger children or used with older teens by adapting the examples and language used.

People often describe anxious feelings as feeling like they are frozen; they can't think, they feel a loss of control, and experience a sense of panic or uncertainty. The De-Ice Your Fears *Express* intervention can be introduced to help children combat that sense of loss of control and unlock their problem-solving and coping skills. The script below will guide you in introducing this Express intervention.

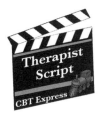

What the Therapist Can Say

"Have you ever been in a car and the windshield was icy? What does the driver do? The driver de-ices the windshield to make it easier to see. When the windshield freezes up, the driver can't see clearly and driving becomes dangerous. Your anxiety is kind of like that. It freezes you up, makes it so you can't see a solution or way to handle things, and that can feel dangerous and scary. We are going to come up with some de-ice statements to help clear up your view and help you more clearly see some ways to cope with difficult situations."

What the Therapist Can Do

The therapist then works with the child and family to identify the thoughts the child has when he or she feels frozen by anxiety—for example, "I'm going to get sick and die"; "I will fail the test"; or "Something bad is going to happen." These thoughts are written on the blurry "frozen" version of the windshield. Once a few frozen thoughts are identified, the therapist should move on so as to be sure and get through the next phase of the intervention. HQ Card 6.4a illustrates an example.

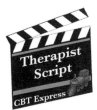

What the Therapist Can Say

"Great job writing down some of your frozen thoughts. There are probably more we haven't listed yet, but you can add those in later as they pop into your head. For now, let's practice de-icing the ones you have written down so far. Those frozen thoughts are keeping you from seeing things clearly and are leaving you feel scared and in danger. When you can't see what's on the other side of the frozen windshield, you can only imagine what is out there, and usually we imagine things more scary than they really are. Let's figure out some de-icing thoughts you can use to melt away the first thought you listed and see what is really on the other side of the windshield."

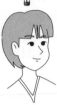

What the Therapist Can Do

The therapist then engages the child in identifying alternative thoughts that will promote coping and decrease catastrophic thinking. Depending on the developmental level, emotional distress, and level of insight of the child, the therapist can use a fill-in-the-blank approach or more detailed evidence testing to identify the new thoughts.

Therapists will not likely have time to introduce and complete detailed evidence testing, and this technique is not designed to do so. Rather, it is meant to start to cast doubt on some of the distorted catastrophic or all-or-nothing thoughts the child is having. Specifically, therapists can present the child with replacement thoughts like "Just because _____, doesn't mean _____," and "Sometimes doesn't mean every time" to start to modify the thought patterns and promote self-talk statements. The therapist can then work with the child to write down some of the specifics on the clear windshield picture on the worksheet, such as "Just because the test is hard doesn't mean I will fail it" or "Sometimes bad things happen, but they don't happen all of the time."

During these exchanges it is important for the therapist to be modeling skills for caregivers during the visits. Therapists should point out to caregivers how they are working with the child to identify the new thoughts, not simply giving them statements to repeat. Therapists should also model praising the child for engaging in the technique and working on the strategy, and can prompt the caregivers to also provide such praise. This is where therapists are required to split their focus. While engaging the child in this activity, therapists can also subtly hold up or tap the Praise block to cue the caregiver to jump in with a reinforcing statement.

Exposure, Exposure, Exposure

Ages: 4 years through teens.

Module: Behavioral Experiments and Exposures.

Purpose: Quickly educate the family on anxiety and the power of exposures.

Rationale: Exposures are extremely powerful in improving anxiety symptoms, but therapists often don't have enough time with families to gradually introduce the concept across multiple sessions.

Materials: Any items to demonstrate exposures (typically things in a clinic or office, including a glove, piece of paper, or pen); HQ Card 6.5, Exposure, Exposure, Exposure (p. 137).

Expected time needed: 15 minutes.

In real estate, "location, location, location" is a mantra used by realtors meaning that neighborhood means everything in the sale of properties. In anxiety treatment, exposure is "everything." Exposure, Exposure, Exposure is a strategy for helping therapists get right to this effective intervention, use exposure techniques to teach families about anxiety, and build a working relationship with families while doing so.

Consider Carmen, who was seen during a well-child visit. Her mother described how she often gets stuck tying and retying her shoes and described other similar patterns of repeating tasks until Carmen believed she had done them "just right." Upon hearing her mother describe these symptoms, Carmen's eyes widened and she moved to the other side of the room. Her mother told the pediatrician she didn't know how to help her daughter. At that point Carmen was clearly listening but pretended to be occupied looking at a picture on the wall. The provider determined psychoeducation would be beneficial to both Carmen and her mother. Knowing exposure work would be helpful, but uncertain as to whether Carmen was ready yet for exposure, the provider took the approach described below and first modeled what exposure was to decrease Carmen's anxiety, and then engaged the family in exposure work. The strategy is described in less than a minute, and then the provider demonstrates the intervention to ensure time does not run out before getting to the crucial step (exposure).

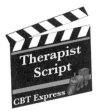

What the Therapist Can Say

"You described a cycle of your child feeling distressed about something, and then doing something that decreases that distress. [*Inserts example from discussion with family, such as 'Carmen feels distress about how she has tied her shoes and reties them until they feel just right.'*]. Repeating the thing that decreases the distress is called a compulsion. It helps people feel better, but only for a short time. Over time, the person needs to do the compulsive behavior more and more just to feel better. To stop this cycle, we help the child experience the distress getting better without completing the compulsive act. I know this might sound confusing, but let me show you what I mean."

At this point, families may have a lot of questions about how this works. Going into a question–answer pattern can certainly be helpful and increase the family's knowledge of the anxiety cycle, obsessive–compulsive disorder (OCD), or phobia patterns, and how exposures work. However, that will take longer than the 15 minutes you may have for intervention, and in the end you will have only talked about the interventions. In *CBT Express*, we recommend teaching by doing. The plan that follows will answer many of the family's questions about exposure by demonstrating what you have just described.

What the Therapist Can Do

We recommend you teach the family about these topics while demonstrating a very simple exposure. Choose an example that may have a pattern that is similar to the child's specific behaviors but different triggers so that the child is less likely to become overly distressed during the modeling. For example, the provider can place a glove or other item on the exam table in a clinic, or a therapist can place a piece of paper on the desk in an office, and introduce exposures using the following 3-minute script.

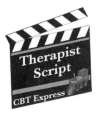

What the Therapist Can Say

"Let's pretend your child feels distressed if a piece of paper is not set down just right on the table. When she sets the paper on the table, she has the urge to pick up the paper and set it down again in a different way, over and over again until it feels just right. When she rearranges the paper, she feels better temporarily, but the more this pattern continues the less control she has over it, and as the pattern strengthens she has to reset the paper more and more often in order to relieve her distress. We want her to learn that the distress will go away if she doesn't rearrange the paper. At first that will be tough, but the more she practices, the easier it will get, and soon the new pattern will be easier. Let me show you what I mean. Let's say you set the paper down [*hands paper to either child or parent*] and it is a little crooked and you want to redo it. And let's say on a scale from 1–10 it feels like you want to redo it at a level 6. And then we wait a while and the feeling starts to fade and it is only a 4. And we wait a little longer and then the urge to move the paper fades more and is only a 2. And then because it is so low, you forget about it and get on with your day. If we practiced that a bunch of times, what do you think would happen?"

Typically at this point the parent or child is able to articulate that eventually the initial rating will be much lower. The therapist continues:

"So we can see that the more you practice something the easier it gets. When it comes to things that are causing you distress, sometimes it is hard to just start not doing the actions or compulsions (like resetting the position of the paper or retying your shoes), so we may have to figure out small steps toward that bigger goal. Anytime a practice feels too hard, always look for the smaller steps to do beforehand and then work up to the part that feels too hard. For example, if setting the paper down was too hard we could have started with just imagining setting the paper down in a crooked way, then we could have had the paper only slightly crooked, and then worked up to more crooked. How do you think we could apply these practice steps to your distress about _____? [*Choose a symptom the family has shared; for Carmen, it could be 'tying your shoes until they feel just right.'*]"

In the next few minutes, the therapist can work with the family to complete at least one exposure and then briefly problem-solve ways to generalize and use the strategies at home. Since providers don't know how many more, if any, opportunities they will have to intervene with the family, every minute has to count, and it is important to get to the intervention early in the interaction with the family.

HQ Card 6.5 can be used with families to outline the Exposure, Exposure, Exposure items completed in the visit, and to identify the next steps that they can continue at home. The small steps should be filled out and completed during the visit, with the larger items being identified for future work either at home or during a future visit.

Exposures are the known "go-to" strategy for OCD and specific phobias, but therapists should also remember that exposure work is effective with other anxiety symptoms as well. Small, spontaneous opportunities for exposure to break anxiety patterns can occur throughout the day. Teaching parents to attend to or create these opportunities will help them use the parenting building blocks previously introduced in Chapter 3 to model and reinforce more adaptive thoughts and problem solving for their anxious child. The following intervention teaches families how to use small opportunities throughout the day as mini-exposures in order to reduce anxiety and promote adaptive coping and problem-solving skills.

Kick Up the Dirt

Ages: Parents of children of all ages.

Module: Behavioral Experiments and Exposures.

Purpose: Use small opportunities throughout the day to model, prompt, and reinforce adaptive responses, coping, and problem solving by anxious youth.

Rationale: Incorporating less anxiety-provoking practices throughout the day will help build the child's skills and confidence in managing his or her emotions in the face of anxiety-producing stimuli.

Materials: Paper and a writing utensil, or a simple task or game (e.g., blocks for stacking).

Expected time needed: 15 minutes.

Kick Up the Dirt is an *Express* technique designed to teach parents strategies for intentionally creating or pointing out small problems throughout the day, and then prompting their children to engage in problem-solving and coping strategies. Creating or identifying "problems" that need solved throughout the day sets up opportunities for practice and success in the use of interventions. These situations serve as mini-exposures to stressors and give children the opportunity to apply newly learned skills to gradually more challenging situations. Parents model, prompt, or reinforce coping and problem solving during these more minor "problems." Doing so multiple times throughout the day can give children increased practice with self-talk, cognitive restructuring, problem solving, and exposures and create more opportunities for success to help with setting new patterns and assist with learning. Therapists can model this during interactions with the family, and then help parents identify potential opportunities to "kick up the dirt" and intentionally challenge their children in small ways throughout the day at home. The following sample script shows how a therapist can introduce the Kick Up the Dirt during a visit with a family.

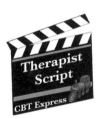

What the Therapist Can Say

"Let's write down one or two worries you had last week that we can work on today. I have a piece of paper here and a pencil. So, what would number one be? [*Try to write a '1' and break the lead of the pencil.*] Uh oh, we have a problem. I just broke the pencil. How can we solve the problem?"

The child will likely say something like "You can use another pencil, or get a pen." Then the therapist can provide specific praise, such as "Good idea. Nice job solving the problem." If the child struggles to come up with a response, a prompt may be needed: "Do you see anything else in the room I could use?"

By labeling this as a "problem" and then using "solve the problem" language, you are starting a verbal script that can be repeated when larger, more challenging problems arise. You are building up examples of successful problem solving with minor issues, and then later parents and children can apply the strategies to more challenging situations. This is essentially graduated exposure to the problems most troubling the child.

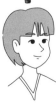

What the Therapist Can Do

This strategy can be applied to many situations. For example, for children with perfectionism symptoms, you can "accidentally" write on the table with a pen while working with the family. Again, the prompt could be something like, "Uh oh, I just wrote on the table with the pen. How can we solve this problem?" The therapist should prompt parents to use this at home—for example, "We ran out of napkins. How can we solve this problem?" (e.g., use paper towels, go to the store, ask a neighbor to borrow some). The therapist can work with families to identify the many opportunities that could occur throughout the day and can model this in the visit.

For example, Isaac, a 9-year-old with attention-deficit/hyperactivity disorder (ADHD), experienced difficulty with transitions due to perfectionism and rigidity. He was drawing while his mother gave the therapist an update on the behavior plan they implemented last week. Isaac looked up at his mother, distraught, when his hand slipped and he got marker on his hand and shirt. The therapist can take this opportunity to prompt Isaac through the use of self-regulation, coping, and problem-solving strategies, while also modeling for Mom how to use these spontaneous situations to promote Isaac's adaptive coping and problem-solving skills.

THERAPIST: Uh oh! We have a problem. You slipped and got marker on your hand and shirt. How can we solve the problem?

ISAAC: I don't know. It's going to be ruined.

THERAPIST: Hmm, you think to yourself, "It is going to be ruined?" and you look like you feel upset. What might help solve the problem when you get something on your hands or shirt?

ISAAC: I don't know.

THERAPIST: Have you ever gotten marker or pen on your hands before?

ISAAC: Yessss.

THERAPIST: And how did you solve the problem when that happened?

ISAAC: It washed off some when I washed my hands and more later when I took my shower.

THERAPIST: So what might happen this time?

ISAAC: I guess the same thing, but what about my shirt?

THERAPIST: So you figured out washing your hands and showering will solve the problem of getting marker off of your hands, good job doing that calmly! Now, what might you try to get the marker out of your shirt?

ISAAC: Mom, will this wash out of my shirt?

THERAPIST: (Holds up the "praise" building block to cue Mom.)

MOM: Isaac, that would be a great way to try and solve the problem! It looks to me like those are the kind of markers that wash out if we use that strong detergent we used when you played that soccer game in the mud and you had grass and mud stains all over your white socks. We can try that when we get home.

THERAPIST: Excellent problem solving. Now what if the marker does not wash out in the laundry?

In the exchange above, the therapist models the approach for Isaac's Mom, prompts her to use the intervention, and then pushes the family to take the problem solving to the next level (e.g., "what if the marker does not wash out?"). This took less than 2 minutes but was

The Praise building block, introduced in Chapter 3, teaches parents to incorporate specific praise into various interactions with their children in order to increase the frequency of desired behaviors. Once the behavioral technique has been taught to parents, therapists can use the block as a nonverbal cue to the parent to praise the behavior they have just observed by their child.

packed full of interventions for Isaac and his mother. Specifically, the family practiced identifying a specific problem, connecting thoughts and feelings, generalizing previously successful solutions, parental prompting and reinforcing of problem solving, and calm self-regulation. The therapist also demonstrated how to take the mini-exposure to the next level by not accepting just one solution for the marked shirt and pushed the family to keep going with a more challenging task.

HQ Card 6.6 provides parents and caregivers with reminders of the Kick Up the Dirt (p. 138) technique and ideas for using it throughout the day during interactions with their children.

It's Like Riding a Bike

Ages: 4 years and older; parents of children/teens.

Module: Psychoeducation; Behavioral Experiments and Exposures.

Purpose: Engage parents and get buy-in for exposure based work and decrease accommodations and avoidance.

Rationale: Parents may inadvertently reinforce the anxiety cycle by rescuing the child from anxiety triggers, avoiding the triggers altogether and therefore sending the message to the child that he or she can't handle the situation.

Materials: Paper and pencil, crayons, or markers.

Expected time needed: 15 minutes.

It's like riding a bike: the more you practice, the easier it gets! This is an important concept for the families with whom we work. Anxiety symptoms can be challenging for children, teens, and their caregivers, and the thought of exposure work can be overwhelming. Family engagement and follow-through with interventions will increase if you are able to help families see that what is difficult in the beginning grows easier with practice. It's Like Riding a Bike is an *Express* strategy designed to illustrate the benefits of repeated practice both on increasing skill level and decreasing distress. Therapists should choose examples based on the child's developmental level. For example, illustrating the benefits of practicing how to tie shoes will be effective for most 9-year-olds, but not applicable for as many 4-year-olds.

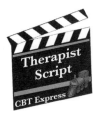

What the Therapist Can Say

"There are lots of things you can do now that you couldn't do when you were younger. What things can you think of that you weren't able to do before but now you can? [*Help the family identify a few things such as riding a bike, tying shoes, walking, or writing one's name.*] That's right, you couldn't do that but then you practiced and practiced and got better and better. When you first started riding a bike, do you think you did it perfectly? No, you wobbled, fell a lot, and maybe even used training wheels. But now you are able to ride your bike without those things! You practiced and practiced and got better and better. The same is true with managing your worries; the more you practice the easier it gets. Here is a worksheet to help list some of the things that are easier for you now that you have practiced them, and there are blank boxes where you can write or draw the things you have not practiced yet and are still difficult."

What the Therapist Can Do

The therapist then works with the family to write or draw examples of things the child can now do after having practiced, as well as a few things related to the treatment goals that he or she is too anxious or "unable" to do at this point. See HQ Card 6.7, It's Like Riding a Bike (p. 139), for an example.

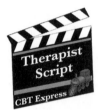

What the Therapist Can Say

"Wow, look at all of the things you practiced that you can now do more easily. And I see some of the things that you struggle with right now. What do you think will happen if you practice one of these things 5 times? 10 times? 100 times? Let's try one now."

The family can continue to add to the list or create a collage of words or pictures. Therapists should encourage parents to identify skills they have been comfortable letting their child practice even if they struggled at first (e.g., walking, dressing themselves, writing their names) and discuss the importance of also practicing skills such as managing emotions, facing fears, and tolerating new situations.

Bridge Building

Ages: 5 years and older.

Module: Behavioral Experiments and Exposures.

Purpose: Create visual representation of a hierarchy and illustrate the steps toward overcoming a specific fear.

Rationale: Exposures and hierarchies are a challenge, and it can be hard for children to understand the systematic approach to overcoming a fear since the thought of the last step prevents them from engaging in the first step.

Materials: Blocks (e.g., Legos), small sticky notes, and a writing utensil.

Expected time needed: 15 minutes.

Bridge Building helps children understand the concept of graduated exposure in a fun and engaging way. Often when exposure is introduced, if a child does not understand the graduated approach, he or she can become overly anxious, shut down, or refuse to engage in the tasks. Bridge Building is an appropriate *Express* exposure technique for when therapists need to go beyond a simple exposure and address in more detail how graduated exposures work. Bridge Building starts with a visual illustration of the approach to engage the child and show the path from current fears to where the child wants to be.

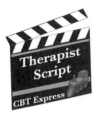

What the Therapist Can Say

"Facing your fears can be hard, but the good news is you don't have to do it all at once. We will take one step at a time starting with where you are now and building a bridge to where you want to be. It is kind of like building a bridge from one spot to another. We start with what you can do pretty easily right now, and each block is one step closer to your goal. Each time you complete a step and overcome a part of your fear, we will add a block like this. We can label each block with what the thing was that you did. We can also add support beams, which are things that can help you be successful, like the support of your parents and your teachers."

What the Therapist Can Do

Therapists should demonstrate how with each exposure another block is added to the bridge. You can label the starting side of the bridge and the "finish" side with what the end goal is (e.g., going to an overnight camp). As with any hierarchy, you will start with easy steps and work up to the harder ones. In contrast to more long-term therapy, with *CBT Express* you may only have a short time to teach and start this concept. Thus, the first several "blocks" should be quickly and easily completed in the *Express* session. If you don't have blocks available, consider cutting pieces of paper and arranging them on a table in the form of a bridge.

Bridge Building was used with 5-year-old Kayli and her mother. Kayli's mother reported that Kayli struggles to separate from her for even short periods of time (e.g., when Mom goes to get the mail). If Kayli is in another room from Mom, she frequently calls out to her, "Where are you?" with a sound of panic in her voice. Mom has delayed sending Kayli to kindergarten as she does not think she can handle the separation. There are few separations that occur throughout the week given the current schedule. These concerns are raised by the family during a primary care visit when discussing starting Kayli in school. The family identifies barriers to engaging in ongoing outpatient psychotherapy, including transportation and child care for other children. A plan is agreed upon to try an *Express* intervention in the clinic and Bridge Building is introduced.

Lego blocks are used to illustrate the approach, first with verbal description and then accompanied by the actual exposures. A common example of skill building is used to illustrate how the approach works. The dialogue below illustrates how, following the initial introduction, the Bridge Building *Express* intervention can be quickly explained and begun.

THERAPIST: (*following introduction above*) Let me show you how this can work. Think about when Kayli learned to walk. She didn't just start walking around the room one day. What did it look like as she learned to walk?

MOM: First she started pulling herself up on furniture, then once she did that a lot she started taking small side steps while holding on to the furniture.

THERAPIST: OK, that is a good example, those would be the first two blocks in the bridge from crawling to walking. (*Connects two blocks.*) What next?

MOM: She started taking the steps holding on with only one hand instead of two, and then she got this push toy and would walk while holding on to that. Then she would let go and just stand there for a minute.

THERAPIST: Excellent description! Those are the next three blocks. (*Adds blocks to the bridge.*) Then what?

MOM: She started taking one or two steps at a time, and then she would fall down and crawl. Then she would take five or six steps, and it just kept building from there.

THERAPIST: (*Adds the additional blocks to the bridge.*) So you see how each "step" built Kayli's skill in walking. We want to approach separating from you the same way. Does that make sense?

MOM: Yeah. I see what you mean. Start with small separations.

THERAPIST: We can start with a few in the clinic today to get started. How does that sound?

MOM: Sure.

This less-than-2-minute example will set the stage for the exposures. The therapist can then work with the family on the initial blocks for separation. For example, the first block could be Kayli and her mom turning so their backs are to each other, and then her mom "hiding" behind the exam curtain in the room. Next Mom or Kayli could step outside of the room briefly and then return, followed by longer separations both in time and distance. Below is an example of how that discussion and practice might go with Kayli and her mother.

THERAPIST: OK, so we will build a bridge from Kayli not tolerating even small separations from you to her being able to cope with regular separations. Kayli, which color block do you want to start with?

KAYLI: Red.

THERAPIST: I like red too. This block is for being able to turn around and face that wall so you can't see Mom sitting here in this chair. How hard to do you think that would be?

KAYLI: Not hard. See!? (*Turns around.*)

THERAPIST: Wow, you stayed so calm and you could not see Mom, but everything was OK. (*In a lower voice to Mom and holding up the Praise block introduced in Chapter 3*) We can use specific praise at each step to reinforce Kayli's efforts and success. Now let's build the next part of the bridge. Kayli, which color block should we use next?

KAYLI: Blue!

THERAPIST: That will look good with the red. For this part of our bridge, how hard would it be if we opened the door to the room, Mom walked out with the door staying opened, and then she walked right back in?

KAYLI: (*more hesitant*) Kinda hard.

THERAPIST: It would be a tougher step. You did so well staying calm when you turned your back to Mom, I bet you can stay calm during this step too. Can we give it a try and see if everything is OK like it was when you turned your back?

KAYLI: I guess.

THERAPIST: (*Makes eye contact with Mom and taps the praise parenting building block.*)

MOM: Kayli you are so brave for trying this! I will be back in the room before you can even blink! (*Walks out of the room and back in.*) Look at that, Kayli, you stayed calm and everything was OK.

THERAPIST: Wow, we have two steps done already on our bridge to success! For the next step, let's have Mom stay out of the room for the count of three.

KAYLI: OK, this one should be the yellow Lego.

THERAPIST: Sounds good.

MOM: (*Leaves the room for the count of three and comes back.*) Wow, Kayli, you are doing amazing at this—you stayed calm again even though it was longer this time.

THERAPIST: You guys are really getting the hang of this. What do you think it would be like to continue these practices at home?

These exposures are completed in about 2 to 3 minutes and prepare the family for the home-based exposures. The therapist then brainstorms with the family when and where they can practice, taking care to point out realistic expectations and how to identify smaller steps if the next one seems too big for Kayli.

Conclusion

Anxiety is a common emotion that can often take hold of a child and quickly become the focus of a therapy visit, primary care visit, or school counseling session. The natural reaction of children and their parents is to avoid anxiety-provoking situations. However, avoidance quickly leads to a pattern of inadvertent reinforcement of anxiety symptoms. Thus, it is important for providers to quickly identify such patterns and be armed with *Express* interventions to reduce the anxiety cycle regardless of the setting. The *Express* interventions in this chapter provide professionals with quick, easy-to-explain interventions that can be utilized in various settings and easily generalized to other environments by families. Using these *Express* interventions can prevent the worsening of anxiety symptoms and provide families with opportunities to combat anxiety.

Don't Sink the Boat

Write your worries on the rocks and then throw them overboard!

Over the River and through the Woods

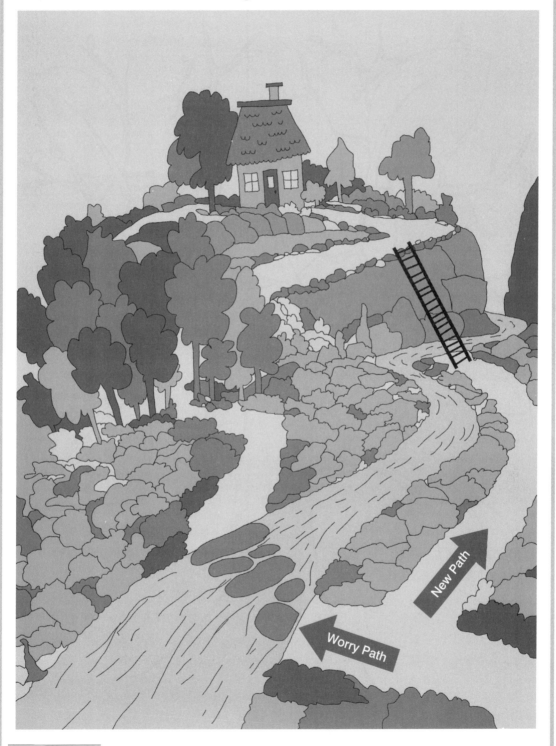

My Worry Tree: Sample

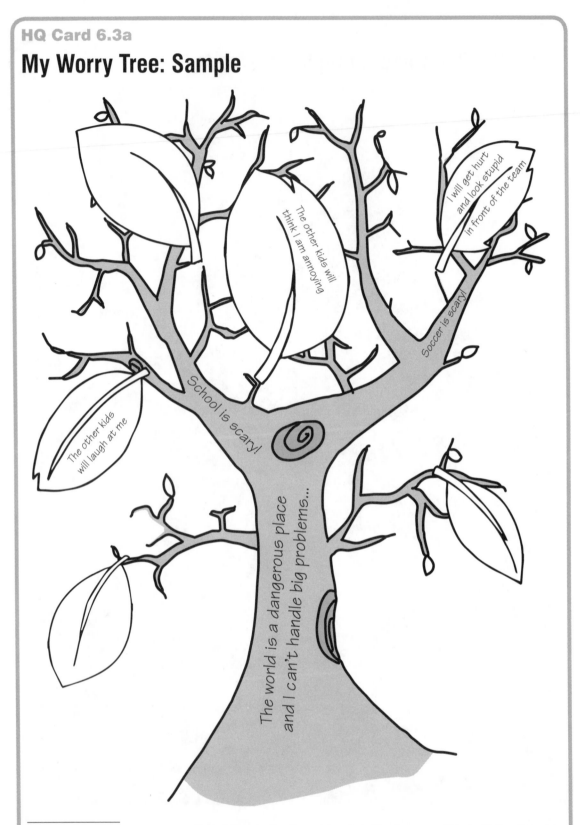

Leaf text: I will get hurt and look stupid in front of the team

Leaf text: The other kids will think I am annoying

Branch text: Soccer is scary!

Leaf text: The other kids will laugh at me

Branch text: School is scary!

Trunk text: The world is a dangerous place and I can't handle big problems...

My Worry Tree

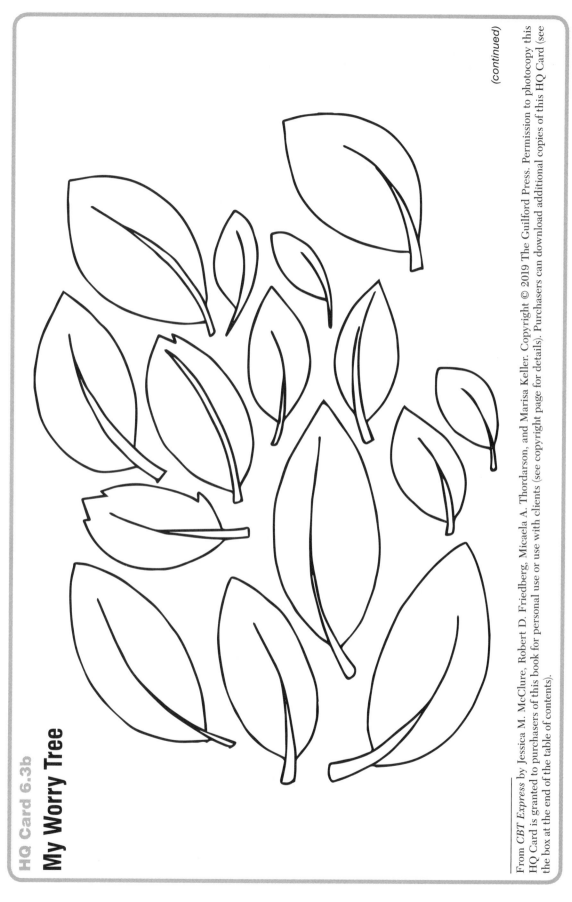

(continued)

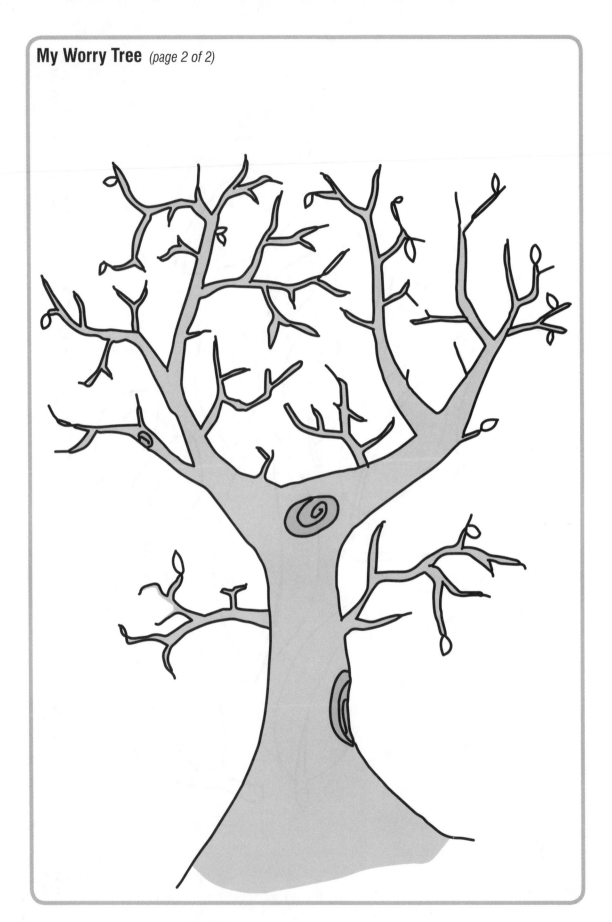

De-Ice Your Fears: Sample

De-Ice (change) your thoughts to melt your worries and remind yourself of ways to cope or solve problems.

I will fail the test.

Something bad is going to happen.

Just because the test is hard doesn't mean I will fail it.

Sometimes bad things happen but they don't happen all of the time.

De-Ice Your Fears

De-Ice (change) your thoughts to melt your worries and remind yourself of ways to cope or solve problems.

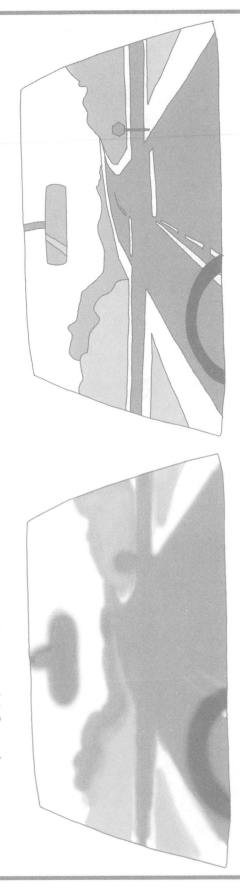

Exposure, Exposure, Exposure

Exposures are extremely powerful in reducing anxiety. Identify and write a small step toward the end goal in each box. Practice each step in order from smallest to biggest. If a step is too challenging, create an in-between box that is more doable.

Kick Up the Dirt

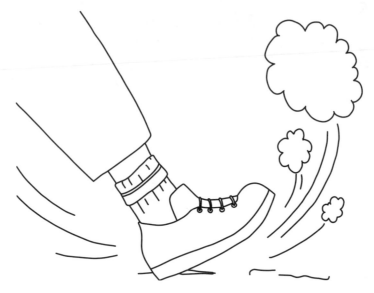

Use small opportunities throughout the day to model, prompt, and reinforce coping and problem solving. Below are some examples. Add ideas you have for using this at home.

✓ Unable to find a pen quickly to write a note.

✓ Favorite clothing item is not clean.

✓ You have run out of preferred food or drink.

✓ Weather interferes with plans.

✓ Something spills while fixing a meal.

✓ You misspell a word while writing a note.

✓ _____.

✓ _____.

✓ _____.

✓ _____.

It's Like Riding a Bike

Circle the things you have already practiced and now can do. Draw or write things you would like to get better at with more practice.

Walking	Being away from Mom overnight
Talking	Going to bed without Mom
Writing my name	
Riding a bike	
Brushing my teeth	
Reading	

CHAPTER 7 ||||||||||||||||||||||||||||||||||||||||||||||||||||||||||||||||

Sadness and Depression

"She doesn't want to do anything except sit in her room watching videos on her phone."

"He's in a bad mood all of the time. A complete grump. It's as if he thinks the world is against him."

"Every little thing gets to him."

"She's so moody. Anything can set her off and she cries over every little thing."

Sadness is a normal feeling that everyone experiences. When the frequency and intensity of sadness increases to the point of interfering with typical daily functioning for children and teens, interventions are needed. Parents or youth sometimes identify the depressive symptoms, or a provider may detect symptoms during the course of a normal office visit. Alternatively, screening measures are becoming more common in pediatric primary care practices, including parental report or youth self-report measures of mood disturbance. In this chapter, we outline *CBT Express* interventions for depressive symptoms that can be quickly implemented in school settings, primary care, or in the context of other treatments once depressive symptoms have been identified.

Brief Statement Regarding Evidence-Based Treatments

The sadness, sluggishness, irritability, withdrawal, and negativity that typically signal depression are directly addressed using cognitive-behavioral strategies. Depression is often maintained by a lack of reinforcement in a child's life coupled with a limited coping repertoire (Spirito, Esposito-Smythers, Wolff, & Uhl, 2011). The more advanced the depression, the more isolated the youth becomes, losing connections to social supports, hobbies, and skills until the youth is tricked into believing there is nothing positive about life. Therefore, CBT tools seek to re-establish a youth's meaningful relationship to their world.

Behavioral interventions involve increasing social interactions, generating opportunities to be successful, and getting the child up and moving to shake off the cobwebs laid on by depression (McCauley, Schloredt, Gudmundsen, Martell, & Dimidjian, 2011). To address rigid, pessimistic thinking, cognitive strategies neutralize negative beliefs, teach problem solving, and encourage flexible, balanced reasoning (Spirito et al., 2011). Studies have shown that completion of homework to generalize skills is a critical aspect in the treatment of depression for youth (Simons et al., 2012). It is the ability to not just acquire but also apply new tools in real-life situations that generates true progress.

CBT demonstrates a host of beneficial outcomes when used to treat symptoms of depression. CBT effectively improves mood, increases functioning, decreases health care utilization costs, and reduces externalizing behavior problems (Arnberg & Ost, 2014; Curry & Wells, 2005; Melvin et al., 2006; March et al., 2004; Weersing et al., 2017). Youth with depression who are treated with CBT take less psychotropic medication in lower doses (Clarke et al., 2005). Importantly, CBT reduces suicidal ideation and alleviates hopelessness in youth with depression (Cox et al., 2012; Melvin et al., 2006; March et al., 2004). Improvements are maintained for at least a year after completion of treatment (Clarke et al., 2005; Kennard, Hughes, & Foxwell, 2016), and intermittent booster sessions prolong effects further (Kennard et al., 2008). CBT effectively treats clinical and subclinical presentations of depression in young patients, and these gains are observed across settings and populations.

CBT is a flexible treatment model that is effective for a wide range of young patients. Research shows that CBT strategies work well regardless of whether delivered in individual, family, or group formats (David-Ferdon & Kaslow, 2008), and are potent in both brief and long-term packages (Stice, Rohde, Seeley, Gau, 2008; Weersing, Jeffreys, Do, Schwartz, & Bolano, 2017). Demographic variables do not affect treatment success (Roselló, Bernal, & Rivera-Medina, 2008; Sandil, 2006; Weersing et al., 2017). Young patients vary widely on factors such as social context, puberty, and executive functioning (factors that may play a role in depression). As a result, developmental sensitivity in treatment design is a particularly important aspect of the therapy (David-Ferdon & Kaslow, 2008; McCauley et al., 2011; Rudolph & Troop-Gordon, 2010). The *CBT Express* interventions included in this chapter allow providers to account for individual patient variation and differences in treatment contexts while preserving the essential elements needed for good care.

Presenting Concerns and Symptoms

Depressive disorders and symptoms are concerning to families and if left untreated can worsen and lead to risky behaviors. Children with depression may present with a range of symptoms, such as sadness, tearfulness, anger, somatic complaints, sleep disturbance, changes in weight, school problems, and substance abuse. Given the variations in presentation, symptoms of depression can be neglected or go undetected by caregivers and providers and can be underreported by children and teens. Additionally, families with competing demands for time and attention may be less likely to pursue treatments. Caregivers may underestimate the severity of symptoms, chalking them up to normal teenage mood swings. Further, teens may feel hopeless about the potential of therapy to help change how they feel. By the very nature of depression, cognitions reflect a lack of hope that things will be better in the future.

Quickly showing the effectiveness of CBT in an *Express* intervention can not only help with the symptoms in the moment, but can lead to increased understanding by families of the potential benefits of CBT. This increased understanding can lead to increased follow-through with future recommendations for treatment interventions or services.

Interventions

Children experiencing sadness or depression are missing out on the joys of childhood. They no longer find previously enjoyable activities fun, and they may therefore withdrawal socially. Often these children demonstrate irritability, and parents observe that they have a quick temper and grumpy disposition. *CBT Express* interventions are not designed to alleviate all depressive symptoms. Rather, these interventions show families that shifts in thoughts and feelings are possible. These interventions are designed to instill hope, and to cast doubt on the permanence of thoughts that children and teens may be experiencing. If families see changes during or following these *Express* interventions, they may be more likely to engage in additional CBT interventions at home or in future treatment, and therefore to further target and improve mood symptoms.

Often a child's or teen's negative self-talk is what parents notice and report to providers in pediatric settings, schools, specialty clinics, or traditional therapy visits. Parents may report that teens are "too hard on themselves" or that they have observed the youth to make negative comments about their appearance, abilities, relationships, or future. Teens too may share or endorse such thoughts when talking to providers, setting the stage for providers to utilize these opportunities to introduce *CBT Express* interventions. The following *Express* interventions target negative cognitions and self-talk statements by teaching the impact of such thoughts and quickly training families on the use of alternative strategies. Teaching self-talk/self-instruction to parents of young children gives parents a way to respond to their youths' negative statements and can set the stage for parents to model, prompt, and reinforce more balanced self-evaluation. Behavioral activation, mood rating, and brief thought-testing techniques can all be addressed with the following *Express* interventions to add to the family's toolbox of strategies for addressing the depressive symptoms.

Pick a Card . . . Any Card

Ages: 6 years and older.

Module: Basic Behavioral Tasks.

Purpose: Increase the child's understanding of the connection between actions and feelings and improve mood through engagement in enjoyable activities.

Rationale: Sad/depressed children and teens make negative predictions about how much fun they will have in activities and they often avoid such activities. Structuring brief, enjoyable activities with feeling ratings before, during and after the activities illustrates the impact of behavioral activation, elevates the mood, and motivates future engagement in such activities.

Materials: Index cards with short activities listed on each card; HQ Card 7.1, Pick a Card . . . Any Card (p. 155).

Expected time needed: 15 minutes.

When children feel sad or depressed, things that used to be fun lack the appeal they used to have for these kids. Depressed youth don't feel interested or motivated to participate in typical childhood activities or events, and they underestimate how much fun they would have if they did engage in the activities. They withdrawal more, engage less, become more lonely and isolated, thus reinforcing their beliefs and sadness. Behavioral activation is an effective way to improve the mood of children and teens by structuring activities that they used to enjoy and then having them rate their moods before, during and after the activities. Pick a Card . . . Any Card helps illustrate the connection between actions and feelings, and can motivate the child to get back to typical childhood activities.

A challenge can be that these children struggle to identify what they "want" to do, often saying "no" to everything or anticipating things will be "boring." The Pick a Card . . . Any Card *Express* intervention provides structure to take that decision making out of the event planning and allows for quick demonstrations in a clinic, school or office environment to promote generalization to home.

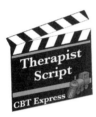

What the Therapist Can Say

"It sounds like you have been spending more time alone and you aren't doing the things that used to be fun for you. You have been feeling down and more alone, and your mom notices you have been crying more often. I have a stack of cards here with different activities on each card. What do you think about trying an experiment? You 'Pick a card . . . Any card' from the stack, rate how you are feeling, and then we will do the activity and re-rate your feelings and see if anything changes."

What the Therapist Can Do

Therapists can have premade cards with simple activities and silly items that can be quickly completed in an *Express* intervention. Next, blank cards can be filled out collaboratively with the family with activities that are realistic for the family to do at home or in the neighborhood. It is important to be mindful of keeping the activities realistic given the family's schedule, financial constraints, or cultural customs and values. Researching free activities available in the community and having a list on hand is recommended. HQ Card 7.1 provides ideas for brief behavioral activation activities that could be written on the cards.

The following example illustrates how a provider uses Pick a Card . . . Any Card with 11-year-old Kristine, who's mom just explained to the provider that Kristine had become more withdrawn and less engaged with school, friends and family after her best friend moved out of state.

THERAPIST: It sounds like you have been spending more time alone and you aren't doing the things that used to be fun for you. You have been feeling down since your best friend moved away. I have a stack of cards here with different activities on each card. What do you think about trying an experiment? You "Pick a card . . . Any card" from the stack, rate how you are feeling, and then we will do the activity and re-rate your feelings and see if anything changes.

KRISTINE: (*Shrugs.*) I guess.

THERAPIST: It is great you are willing to give it a try. Here are the cards, just pick any card.

KRISTINE: (*Selects a card from the stack and reads it to herself, then grins.*)

THERAPIST: You are grinning. What does the card say?

KRISTINE: "Play Simon Says with your parent." I think Mom is going to say no way.

MOM: I will do it!

THERAPIST: OK, Kristine—you are Simon. But before we start, from 0–10 how are you feeling right now, with 10 being as happy as you can possibly be and 0 being no happiness and totally down or depressed?

KRISTINE: I am like a 2, I guess. I feel blah but it isn't a zero like the end of the world or anything.

THERAPIST: OK, Simon, start when you are ready!

KRISTINE: Simon says clap your hands. Simon says touch your head. Simon says stand up.

MOM: (*doing all the items*) Wow, you are going fast, but I am keeping up!

KRISTINE: Sit down.

MOM: Nope, you aren't tricking me!

KRISTINE: OK, fine. Simon says balance on one foot.

MOM: (*balancing for a minute then starting to wobble*)—Kristine!

KRISTINE: Simon says keep balancing! (*smiling*)

MOM: Ohhhhhh, woooaaaaaa. (*Loses her balance and flops back into the chair laughing.*) You got me! I have terrible balance.

KRISTINE: (*Laughs.*) That's OK, Mom, you tried.

THERAPIST: I see you laughing and smiling. I wonder what your rating is right now.

KRISTINE: Huh I guess it is more like a 4 or 5 now. It was kind of funny to see Mom try and do that.

THERAPIST: So it was a 2 before the game, and then jumped all the way to a 4 or 5 in about 2 minutes! That is amazing, you really used the Pick a Card to change your actions and then change your mood! Imagine what will happen if you play games like this several times a week at home. Now, let's talk about what things could get in the way of doing this at home so you will be ready for what could come up when you play Pick a Card at home.

The therapist used praise for Kristine's engagement in the activity, gave an appropriate amount of direction and instruction, and then sat back and let the parent and child practice together. Following the game, the therapist helps Kristine rerate her feelings and then ties the results of the game to the future showing Kristine's control to change her feelings. The therapist then quickly transitions to setting up the home practices to be sure the success will be built upon. The entire exchange took less than 10 minutes and leaves plenty of time for setting up the homework and discussing how to create additional cards to use at home.

Echo . . . Echo . . . Echo . . .

Ages: 6 years and older; parents of children of all ages.

Module: Cognitive Restructuring.

Purpose: Teach families the impact of negative self-talk and how to quickly modify self-talk statements to reduce the reinforcement of negative thoughts about self, others and the future.

Rationale: Increasing the understanding of the connection between thoughts and feelings can help children and teens be more aware of what they are saying to themselves. Increasing parental awareness of this connection can provide opportunities for parents to model, prompt and reinforce more balanced self-talk by their children.

Materials: HQ Card 7.2, Echo . . . Echo . . . Echo . . . (p. 156), and a writing utensil.

Expected time needed: 10 minutes.

Children are faced with daily stressors at home and school. Family conflict, financial instability, parental mental health issues, as well as the demands of school work, bullying at school, or peer conflict can be interpreted by a child or teen as insurmountable and permanent stressors. Echo . . . Echo . . . Echo demonstrates the impact of negative self-talk when facing such stressors and sets the stage for modifying thoughts. What is said by the youth (either aloud or in her head) bounces back like an echo repeating the statement and reinforcing the negative thought. The echo concept is used to explain to families that if the child (and/ or parent) reduces negative thoughts and increases more balanced "echo" thoughts, emotions can be impacted in a positive way. This strategy plants the seed for future cognitive restructuring by giving quick strategies for changing the thoughts from negative to more helpful. Using the "more helpful" term rather than "positive" or "true" when describing the new thoughts also avoids a lengthy debate about the accuracy of the original "echo" thoughts. Providers should not debate with the child about whether his thoughts are true or not, but rather need to help the child focus on whether the current thoughts are *helpful* in improving his mood. If the thoughts are determined *not* to be helpful, then the focus can be shifted to more helpful thoughts/statements.

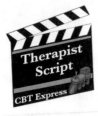

What the Therapist Can Say

"When you yell something into a cave or canyon, it will echo back the sound or word that you shouted. The same happens with things you say to yourself. If you tell yourself you are stupid, ugly, unliked . . . [*insert examples the family has shared about what the child says to himself*] then your brain basically echoes that back to you. The more you say it, the more it echoes, and the more down you feel. We want to stop the echo and help you take control of changing the things you don't like. If you 'shout' more helpful statements, then the echoes will also be more helpful. More helpful echoes can improve how you are feeling and make it easier to get back to doing the things you used to enjoy, like spending time with friends."

What the Therapist Can Do

The therapist can use HQ Card 7.2 to illustrate this concept with the family and help the family start to identify replacement self-talk statements. Reminding the family of the Praise building block is helpful too.

Parents can praise the child's engagement in the intervention as well as use of the Echo technique at home. The technique should be practiced with the family during the visit, and then a brief discussion for use at home can help set up follow-through with practicing outside of the visit.

Written in Stone

Ages: 8 years and older and parents.

Module: Cognitive restructuring.

Purpose: Teach families that feelings and thoughts are transient and can and will change in the future.

Rationale: When children are depressed they believe they will feel that way forever and that things will not change. This intervention illustrates that thoughts and feelings can and will change and that very few things are "set in stone."

Materials: HQ Cards 7.3a and 7.3b, Written in Stone, sample and blank cards (pp. 157–158), and a writing utensil.

Expected time needed: 10 minutes.

Written in Stone is an *Express* intervention that can quickly demonstrate that thoughts and feelings change and recognizing this can help children cope with the intensity of the moment when feeling depressed. This strategy shines a light on the vast number of things that are changeable, like thoughts and feelings, and how few things never change (e.g., they are set or written in stone). See the therapist script (What the therapist can say) and the following dialogue, which illustrates completing this *Express* intervention with Kyle and his mother.

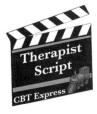

What the Therapist Can Say

"Have you ever heard the expression, 'written in stone'? People often use that to describe something that won't change. Sometimes people use that expression to emphasize that something *will* change but specifically saying it is '*not* written in stone.' When someone is feeling down or depressed, that person often views thoughts and feelings as being 'written in stone' which can add to feeling hopeless that things will ever change. But in fact, very few things are unchanging or set in stone. Let's try something to show what things are and are not 'written in stone.' As fast as you can, I would like you and your mom to use this worksheet to list things about you that have changed since you were born—for example your height or how much you sleep. These things are not written in stone—they change. OK, great, that is quite a list. Now, what things have not changed? It seems like it is a lot harder for you to list things that have not changed. What do you think that means?"

THERAPIST: We have been talking about how sad and down you have been feeling, Kyle.

KYLE: Yeah, I guess.

THERAPIST: Now I would like to try something called Written in Stone and see if it makes a difference in how you feel.

KYLE: I guess.

THERAPIST: You mentioned a moment ago that things suck and you know they will always suck. That sounds like it won't change. What I want you to do now is focus on the things that have changed in the past for you.

KYLE: OK.

THERAPIST: As fast as you can, I would like you and your mom to use this worksheet to list things about you that have changed since you were born—for example your height or how much you sleep.

(Kyle and his mom work on the list for 2 minutes, generating a lot of examples.)

THERAPIST: OK, great, that is quite a list. Now, what things have not changed?

(Kyle and his mom struggle to identify many items.)

THERAPIST: It seems like it is a lot harder for you to list things that have not changed. What do you think that means?

KYLE: More stuff in life changes than doesn't I guess.

THERAPIST: Now let's circle the things that are considered feelings.

KYLE: *(Circles "how cold I feel," "how tired I am," "how sad I was when my dog died," "how upset I was about my algebra grade.")*

THERAPIST: Those are all types of feelings, nice work. Now, which list did you put all four of those on?

KYLE: They are all on the change side. They all changed as time went by.

THERAPIST: Exactly, you are seeing the pattern. Feelings actually do change. And are there any feelings on the "don't change" list?

KYLE: No—I could only come up with a few things on that list. Fingerprints was already there, and that made me think of DNA which we learned about in bio so I added that. I also put "who my mom is" because she will always be my mom even when I grow up.

THERAPIST: You noticed how much more difficult it was to come up with "don't change" things, and with the "change" list we stopped while you were still writing so you probably could have come up with even more. How might realizing this help you when you are feeling like "things suck and you know they will always suck"?

KYLE: I guess I could remind myself that is a feeling and it will change at some point even though it feels like it won't.

THERAPIST: That is a great self-talk statement. We can also try some other strategies to address those "sucky" feelings (if time, therapist could then introduce *Pick a Card* at this visit or a future visit depending on the setting and amount of time with the family).

What the Therapist Can Do

If the family struggles to identify items for the lists, the therapist can name things and have the child or teen label whether they have changed in the past or will change in the future. For example, the therapist might say, "your favorite movie" or "how hungry you are" and the child responses "change" or "don't change" and adds it to the list. The therapist then could say something like, "what about your height? Has that changed or stayed the same?" The therapist should then work with the family to write down the items on HQ Card 7.3b. Kyle's sample (HQ Card 7.3a) demonstrates how the therapist and Kyle's family filled this out during the visit.

Defeating the Negative Thought Troll

Ages: 8–12 years.

Module: Cognitive Restructuring.

Purpose: Replace the irritating self-damning thoughts with more accurate private speech.

Rationale: Depressed youth experience self-critical and at times self-loathing thoughts that decrease their sense of self-efficacy, worthiness, attractiveness, and competence.

Materials: HQ Cards 7.4a and 7.4b, Defeating the Negative Thought Troll, sample and blank cards (pp. 159–160), and a writing utensil.

Expected time needed: 10 minutes.

Trolls are ugly and irritating creatures who keep out of sight and live in dark places such as caves or under bridges. More recently, trolls are seen as individuals who post negative, argumentative, and bothersome messages on social media platforms. Negative thoughts are similar to these trolls. They emerge out of the darkness to bug young patients with their irritating, condemning, and often ugly messages.

Defeating the Negative Thought Troll is a self-instructional method that facilitates cognitive restructuring. It teaches young patients to talk back to this private bully. The task is very simple. In Step 1, the therapist teaches the patient about trolls. Step 2 involves writing down the troll thought. In Step 3, the patient creates a coping thought that quiets down the trolling. These straight forward steps can be completed in 10 minutes during a clinic visit, with a school counselor during a free period, or in the context of a traditional therapy visit.

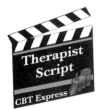

What the Therapist Can Say

THERAPIST: Brandon, do you know what a troll is?

BRANDON: Hmm . . . I think so . . . They are kinda like monsters . . . They are ugly.

THERAPIST: And they really bug people too, right?

BRANDON: I think so.

THERAPIST: So in that way, they are like the ugly things you say to yourself when you are feeling down. The thoughts are like trolls. Does that make sense?

BRANDON: I guess.

THERAPIST: I have this worksheet I want to share with you. (*Takes out HQ Card 7.4a*). On this side, where you see the troll, is where the negative thoughts go. Look down here. What are the things that are written down?

BRANDON: "I am ugly," "I am stupid," "No one will be my friend."

THERAPIST: How close are they to what goes through your head?

BRANDON: Pretty close.

THERAPIST: On the other column, we have to come up with a way to defeat this irritating troll. On the worksheet, there are some examples. What was said back to the troll?

BRANDON: Umm, for I'm stupid, "Forget you, Troll! You don't know me. I know me. Stupid is just name-calling. I am more than that!" and for I'm ugly, "Go back in your hole troll, you only come out when I am sad."

THERAPIST: So what do you think about those come backs?

BRANDON: They might work.

THERAPIST: Good. Are there ways you could make them stronger?

BRANDON: No, they are OK, I guess.

THERAPIST: Look, here is one that does not have a comeback. Let's see if you can come up with one.

BRANDON: Umm. STUFF IT, TROLL! You don't even know who is my friend. You cannot say that!

THERAPIST: Good comebacks. So for homework, how willing are you to write down your own troll thoughts and comebacks to defeat them on this worksheet?

In less than 10 minutes the therapist has taught Brandon to defeat the negative thought troll. In addition, the therapist has given Brandon the opportunity to successfully practice the strategy during the interaction. The therapist then concludes by engaging Brandon in planning the therapy homework completion to increase the likelihood that Brandon will use this strategy at home and school.

Shake It Off

Ages: 8–14 years.

Module: Cognitive Restructuring.

Purpose: Replace the depressogenic private speech with more productive alternatives.

Rationale: Depressed youth are challenged with negative views of self, others, their experiences, and the future. Shake It Off provides the opportunity to counter these debilitating thoughts with coping responses.

Materials: "Shake It Off" song, sticky notes, HQ Card 7.5, Shake It Off (p. 161), and a writing utensil.

Expected time needed: 10–15 minutes.

Shake It Off is a very fast and fun way to conduct self-instruction with youth. The procedure makes use of the popular Taylor Swift song "Shake It Off" and basic self-instructional techniques. The method begins with writing young patients' negative thoughts on post-it sticky notes. The therapist also writes some negative thoughts on the sticky notes as well. After the thoughts are recorded, patients and therapists each stick the notes on their arms and hands. Next, the therapist explains, "You know the Taylor Swift song, 'Shake It Off'? Well, it is going to help us get rid of your negative thoughts and replace them with coping thoughts. Let's see how we do it."

The song is played and when the child hears the chorus (e.g., "*haters gonna hate, hate, hate, hate, hate. Baby, I'm just gonna shake, shake, shake, shake, shake. I shake it off, I shake it off*"), he or she is instructed to flap his or her arms to shake off the negative thoughts. After patients shed the negative thoughts, the sticky notes are picked up and new coping thoughts that counter the distressing thoughts are developed. Patients then stick the new thoughts to the back of the old one to create coping cards. The following dialogue illustrates how Kelly used Shake It Off with her therapist.

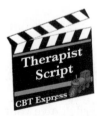

What the Therapist Can Say

THERAPIST: OK, Kelly, I remember that you are a big Taylor Swift fan. Well, we are going to use one of her songs to get rid of some of your negative thoughts. How does that sound?

KELLY: I am a *real* Swifty!

THERAPIST: Wonderful. First, take these sticky notes and write down the things that go through your mind when you are feeling sad and worried. I'll write some too. *(They write down the thoughts)*

Now let's stick them on our hands and arms. Next, we are going to listen to the song and when Taylor sings the words "shake it off," we're going to shake off the thoughts (demonstrates by jumping around and flapping arms). Do you think you can do that?

KELLY: Sure.

(The song is played.)

THERAPIST: That was fun! Next, let's pick up the thoughts and see if we can change them so they don't make you feel sad or worried. We'll write them down and stick them back-to-back so whenever you think things like, "I can't do anything right," you have something to quiet them down.

What the Therapist Can Do

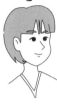

This is a very active exercise so we recommend therapists be animated and enthusiastic. Jumping around and vigorously shaking off the sticky notes is strongly encouraged. The exercise can be repeated several times. It is also important that the discarded thoughts are replaced with alternatives. These alternate thoughts should include an active coping component. HQ Card 7.5 can be used to generate ideas for the sticky notes.

Fox Talk

Ages: 8–14 years.

Module: Cognitive Restructuring.

Purpose: Develop a way to translate or transform inaccurate internal messages into more accurate appraisals.

Rationale: Depressed youth are prone to various distortions which skew their interpretations of external and internal events.

Materials: Song, video, or book version of "What Does the Fox Say?," HQ Cards 7.6a and 7.6b, Translating Fox Talk, sample and blank cards (pp. 162–163), and a writing utensil.

Expected time: 10–15 minutes.

Similar to Shake It Off, Fox Talk is a self-instructional task that makes use of popular culture. The popular song of a few years ago, "What Does the Fox Say?" created by Ylvis, provides the platform for launching this fast-paced exercise. Fox Talk teaches children that many negative automatic thoughts are illogical, distorted, and inaccurate. For instance, the song lyrics begin, "Dog goes woof, cats go meow, bird goes tweet, and the mouse goes squeak. Cow goes moo, frog goes croak, and elephant goes toot." However, when it comes to the fox, the fox says, "ring-ding-ding-ding, dinger-ringed-ding." While all the descriptions of animals are accurate up to this point, "ring-ding-ding-ding, dinger-ringed-ding" is clearly inaccurate and illogical. Therefore, the next task is to correct the fox talk.

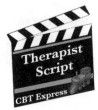

What the Therapist Can Say

THERAPIST: Matilda, do you know the song "What Does the Fox Say?"

MATILDA: I haven't heard that song in a long time.

THERAPIST: Would it be OK if we watch the video? (*Plays video.*)

MATILDA: It's kind of silly.

THERAPIST: Yeah, we have to translate or change the fox talk into things that make more sense. We know the "dog goes woof, cats go meow, bird goes tweet, and the mouse goes squeak. Cow goes moo, frog goes croak, and elephant goes toot." And the fox doesn't really say "ring-ding-ding-ding, dinger-ringed-ding." The fox talk is jibber jabber or speech that really does not make sense. Our job is to change what is not true to something that fits the facts better. How does that sound?

MATILDA: I'm not sure. What do I have to do?

THERAPIST: Take a look at the Fox Talk worksheet [HQ Card 7.6a]. On this side, we have the fox jibber jabber. Can you read the thoughts there?

MATILDA: "I will never get good grades" and "Everyone hates me."

THERAPIST: Matty, do *you* ever have thoughts like that?

MATILDA: I do.

THERAPIST: OK, so what we have to do is translate the jibber jabber into something more understandable. It's kind of like what you do when you translate for your *abuelos*. The way we translate the fox talk is with these hints, like replacing words like *always, never, all, none, everyone, everything, nothing, must, will,* and *should* with *sometimes, some, kind of, maybe, might, could,* and so on. How does that sound?

MATILDA: I think I get it.

THERAPIST: OK. Let's try one. How can you use the hints to translate the Fox talk that says, "I will never get good grades."

MATILDA: Hmm . . . Maybe "I probably will get mostly good grades, but I might get a bad grade if the work is too hard."

THERAPIST: That is a good start. Now let's try one of your own Fox Talk messages.

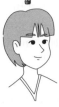

What the Therapist Can Do

The therapist begins the exercise by playing the video or audio recording of "What Does the Fox Say?" We recommend that therapists emphasize and or amplify the silliness inherent in the song. Therapists might add funny gestures as well. When the sample worksheet is presented, make sure you work to personalize and individualize it. This active and engaging *Express* intervention will be memorable for the child, and he or she can easily be prompted by parents at home to continue to work on self-instruction.

Guardians of Your Brain

Ages: 8–14 years.

Module: Cognitive Restructuring.

Purpose: Construct a self-protective process which shields young patients from painful self-recriminations.

Rationale: Guardian of Your Brain helps insulate young patients from the intrusive self-recriminations and pessimistic predictions that invade their private speech.

Materials: HQ Card 7.7, Guardians of Your Brain (p. 164), and a writing utensil.

Expected time needed: 10–15 minutes.

Guardians of Your Brain is a self-instructional technique that wards off the negative thoughts that attack young patients. Negative thoughts are seen as invaders who are engaging in a hostile takeover of young patients' inner lives. The Guardian protects the brain against the attacker by offering a variety of strategies. Based on the answer to the strategic questions, a battle plan is created.

In Step 1, patients and therapists record their "mind attacker" ("I'm so lame"; "No one will be my friend"). Next, patients' attention is directed toward the six Guardian strategies. They then select and note the strategies that protect them from this predatory thought. The last step is based on the strategy they selected. That strategy is used by patients to construct a battle plan to defend themselves against pernicious beliefs.

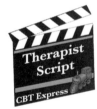

What the Therapist Can Say

TARIK: My thoughts are so painful. It is like my brain is sticking me with swords.

THERAPIST: I bet it does feel like you are under attack. You need a guardian of your brain to keep out the thoughts that stab you.

TARIK: Yeah! Where do I find something like that?

THERAPIST: (*Smiles.*) Funny you should ask. I have this worksheet right here called Guardians of Your Brain [HQ Card 7.7]. Take a look.

TARIK: I like the guy on the front. How do I use it?

THERAPIST: I'll show you. First, let's write down the painful thought that was attacking you.

TARIK: I'll never do as well in school as my sister. I'm a total lost cause. My brain is filled with stinky garbage.

THERAPIST: Wow. That thought really winds you. Let's try out some guardian strategies, OK? Read over these tips and see if there is something there that could protect you.

TARIK: Hmm. The one that says, "Is this thought harmful or helpful to me?" And "Is the attacker thought making me see only the worst in myself?"

THERAPIST: Great! Let's write these in the column below. Now, how can we build a battle plan based on the answers to the question "Is this helpful to you?"

TARIK: NO! It just makes me feel bad.

THERAPIST: OK. Let's write that down. This mind attacker thought only makes me feel bad. Now the second question: "Is the thought only making you seeing the worst in yourself?"

TARIK: Yes!

THERAPIST: OK. So the mind attacker is only trying to make you see the worst in yourself and nothing else. So should you believe a thought that only makes you see the worst in yourself and makes you feel bad?

TARIK: No, I guess not.

THERAPIST: Now read over this battle plan we just wrote down together.

TARIK: My mind attacker just makes me feel bad and is trying to make me see the worst in myself and nothing else. I do not have to believe a thought like that.

THERAPIST: Do you think it would be helpful to write this on an index card and read it over whenever you get a mind attack like you are stinky garbage and a lost cause?

What the Therapist Can Do

Using HQ Card 7.7 or an index card during this *Express* intervention provides the depressed child with a quick and effective intervention to begin to change thoughts in the moment, while also providing a cue (index card) to prompt cognitive restructuring at later times too. By using the metaphor, the therapist helps increase the chances the child will recall the strategy later. This approach can also increase the child's engagement and willingness to talk about thoughts and feelings during and following the intervention.

Conclusion

Depressive symptoms are a challenging clinical presentation for many providers, and there are often numerous barriers to depressed children getting ongoing traditional CBT for depression. By implementing one or more of these *Express* interventions at the point of identification of symptoms, providers can engage the family, demonstrate the effectiveness of the CBT approach, and increase the likelihood of follow-through with future recommendations. Since the interventions are quickly completed in less than 15 minutes, they can easily be introduced and completed in a primary care clinic, school counselor's office, or other settings where providers are interacting with children. Physically demonstrating and practicing the techniques with the family are necessary for maximum effectiveness. By using the 10–15 minutes to really engage the family in the *Express* techniques, the provider is directly impacting the depressive symptoms in real time and setting the stage for future improvement.

Pick a Card . . . Any Card

On one side of the card, write activities that can be completed quickly during the *Express* session. After demonstrating the intervention with the family, have them create additional cards with things that can be completed easily at home or in their community. The child can draw pictures or designs on the cards to make them more colorful.

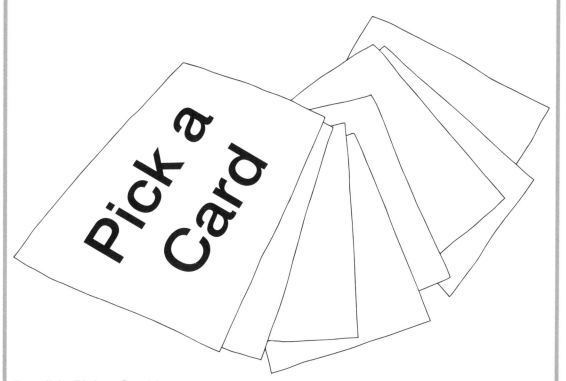

Possible Pick-a-Card items:

1. Play Simon Says (this gets the heart rate up and children can find it silly, particularly if parents and providers play with them).

2. Watch a funny YouTube video (providers should have developmentally appropriate videos ready).

3. Tell a silly joke.

4. Demonstrate a magic trick or show a video of a magic trick.

Echo . . . Echo . . . Echo . . .

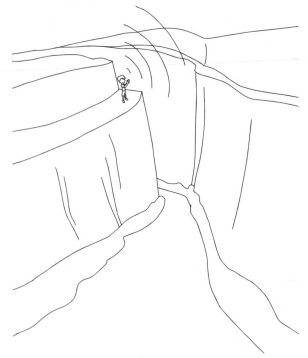

What thoughts are you currently shouting to yourself that are then echoing back to you?

_____

_____

_____

_____

_____

What new thoughts can you try to echo?

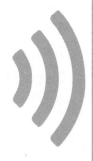

_____

_____

_____

_____

_____

Written in Stone: Sample

Some things don't change, but most things do change. When we confuse changeable things (like feelings) with things that aren't able to be changed, we can feel more sad, down, or depressed. We treat our negative thoughts or feelings as if they are *written in stone* and will never change. See if you can list things in the change or don't change categories. Fingerprints and feelings are done for you. Add as many as you can think of in 2 minutes.

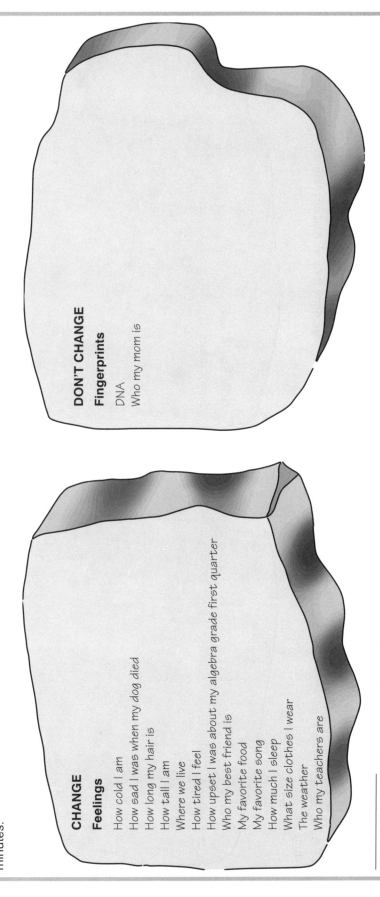

DON'T CHANGE

Fingerprints

DNA

Who my mom is

CHANGE

Feelings

How cold I am
How sad I was when my dog died
How long my hair is
How tall I am
Where we live
How tired I feel
How upset I was about my algebra grade first quarter
Who my best friend is
My favorite food
My favorite song
How much I sleep
What size clothes I wear
The weather
Who my teachers are

Written in Stone

Some things don't change, but most things do change. When we confuse changeable things (like feelings) with things that aren't able to be changed, we can feel more sad, down, or depressed. We treat our negative thoughts or feelings as if they are *written in stone* and will never change. See if you can list things in the change or don't change categories. Fingerprints and feelings are done for you. Add as many as you can think of in 2 minutes.

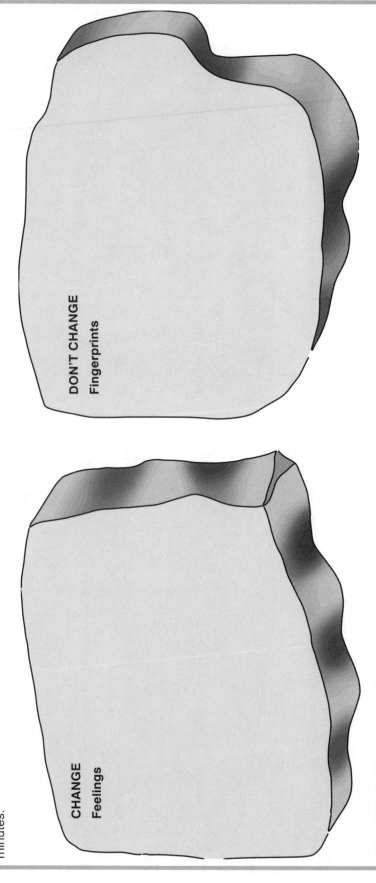

DON'T CHANGE
Fingerprints

CHANGE
Feelings

Defeating the Negative Thought Troll: Sample

What your troll says 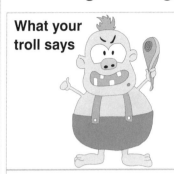	What I say to defeat the troll 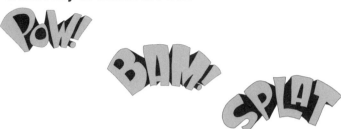
I am ugly.	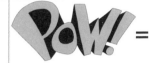 = Go back in your hole, Troll. You only come out when I am sad.
I am stupid.	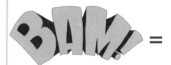 = Forget you, Troll! You don't know me. I know me. Stupid is just name calling. I am more than that!
No one will be my friend.	SPLAT = Stuff It, Troll! You don't even know who is my friend. You cannot say that!

Defeating the Negative Thought Troll

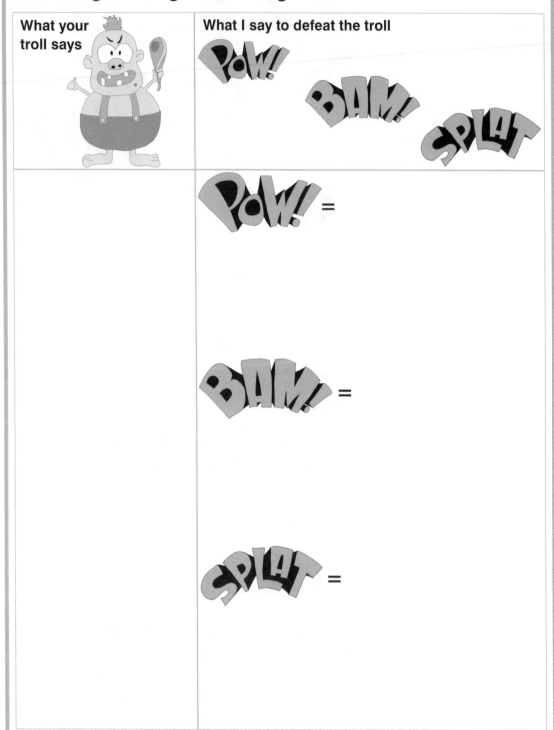

What your troll says	What I say to defeat the troll
	POW! =
	BAM! =
	SPLAT =

Shake It Off

Practice coming up with Shake It Off thoughts to answer the negative thoughts going through your head.

Sticky Note Thought → Shake It Off Thought

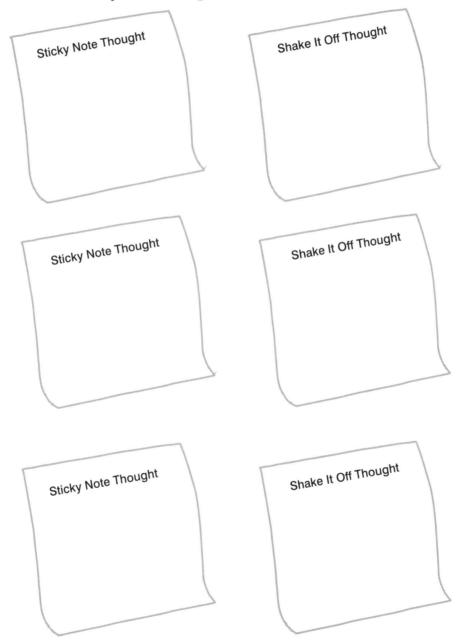

Sticky Note Thought | Shake It Off Thought

Sticky Note Thought | Shake It Off Thought

Sticky Note Thought | Shake It Off Thought

Translating Fox Talk: Sample

Your Fox says:	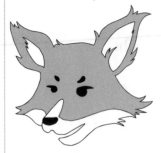 **Your translation=** Hint: Change words like *always, never, all, none, everyone, everything, nothing, must, will,* and *should* to *sometimes, some, kind of, maybe, might, could,* and so on.
I will never get good grades.	I probably will get mostly good grades, but I might get a bad grade if the work is hard to do.
Everyone hates me.	Some kids don't like me, but some kids do.

Translating Fox Talk

Your Fox says:	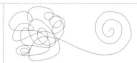
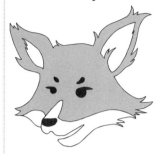	**Your translation=** Hint: Change words like *always, never, all, none, everyone, everything, nothing, must, will,* and *should* to *sometimes, some, kind of, maybe, might, could,* and so on.

Guardians of Your Brain

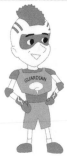

Mind Attackers	Guardian Strategies:	Mind's Battle Plan
	1. Be careful—even though attacker thoughts seem true at first, they may be false. 2. Is this thought helpful or harmful to myself or others? 3. Is the attacker thought trying to trick me? 4. Is the attacker thought trying to make me do something that will build me up or tear me down? 5. Is the attacker thought making me see ONLY the worst in myself, others, or the situation? 6. Are strong feelings making these thoughts seem more true than they are?	

Medical Nonadherence

"She can't swallow pills."

"It's too hard to get him to do it."

"We're so busy—we just forget."

"It's not working!"

Health behaviors are important practices that are not always taken into consideration as treatment targets for youth. However, variations in adherence to medical regimens produce a wide range of long-term outcomes. Children and adolescents who fail to follow regimens use more medication, access health care services with greater frequency, visit urgent cares and emergency departments more often, and experience many more negative consequences (Christopherson & Mortweet, 2013; Roberts, Aylward, & Wu, 2014). There is no uniform definition of medical nonadherence. Medical regimens are composed of a wide range of behaviors. This makes it difficult to establish what degree of noncompliance merits designation as nonadherence. For the purposes of this chapter, nonadherence refers generally to a failure to follow recommendations that renders treatment less effective.

Nonadherence can be a result of numerous barriers to adherence. Parents and children may be frustrated by psychosocial barriers, they may struggle to understand complex treatment regimens, and they may deem expectations unrealistic. Medical providers sometimes perceive families as resistant, willful, confused, or inconsistent (Roberts et al., 2014). We need to keep in mind that families and physicians share a common goal: to address the medical concern. Nonadherence is rarely deliberate or intentional, and often emerges from a failure to effectively communicate. Families and physicians approach problems from two distinct perspectives: the family system and the medical model. Families do not understand all the pieces of the problem (e.g., why it arose, how it can be prevented in the future, how to treat it, what the long-term prognosis is, how treatment can help and how it can't, what will the child be at risk for if the issue is not treated now). The physician or medical provider may not grasp the various real-life factors that affect compliance (e.g., school schedules, extracurricular activities, home life, cultural factors, siblings, work). Behavioral health aims to bridge the gap between these perspectives, paving a path to mitigate barriers and improve adherence (Rapoff, 2010).

The *CBT Express* interventions in this chapter will help providers and families address barriers and increase compliance with minimal investment and maximal gain. Behavioral health clinicians positioned in primary care settings and multidisciplinary clinics can use these interventions in the context of broader treatment. Pediatricians, nurses, care managers, and technicians may also benefit from using these interventions to address problems with following medical recommendations. Psychiatrists, residents, and other medical providers working with families in inpatient or outpatient care clinics can incorporate these interventions into their practice to enhance compliance.

The following *CBT Express* interventions address the three most prevalent medical noncompliance issues: pill-swallowing difficulties, medication nonadherence, and nutrition plan nonadherence. At the end of each main topic, a troubleshooting guide is included to instruct providers on how to modify interventions in the face of the most frequent complications.

Brief Statement Regarding Evidence-Based Treatments

Research shows CBT effectively addresses medical nonadherence (Cortina, Somers, Rohan, & Drotar, 2013; Hankinson & Slifer, 2013). Most medical regimen noncompliance requires short-term, problem-focused intervention drawing from discrete modules of CBT, rather than complete protocols. To maximize compliance, clinicians first must ensure a true understanding of what is prescribed by the medical provider. Clear and concrete psychoeducation may be sufficient to address nonadherence (Weersink, Taxis, McGuire, & van Driel, 2015). Objective data gathered in the course of target monitoring are required to assess outcomes and determine how to intervene (Cortina et al., 2013). In most cases, problem solving, contingency plans, and other behavioral interventions lead to improvements in compliance with medical regimens (Luersen et al., 2012; Modi, Guilfoyle, & Rausch, 2013; Wu et al., 2013).

At times, parent and child beliefs interfere with compliance, and thus cognitive interventions are required to address these internal barriers (McGrady, Ryan, Brown, & Cushing, 2015). Exposures create critical learning experiences for children and their parents, teaching that adherence is feasible (Meltzer et al., 2006; Schiele et al., 2014). Treatment of medical nonadherence emphasizes the assessment of the challenges the family faces, then involves the direct and specific dismantling of the identified obstacles. Overall, the evidence in support of cognitive-behavioral strategies to treat medical noncompliance provides a clear rationale for use of the following *CBT Express* interventions.

In the film *Mary Poppins*, the protagonist sang, "In every job that must be done, there is an element of fun." However, when a spoonful of sugar is not inherent to the task, a sweet enhancement may be indicated. Medical regimens are typically important for long-term prognosis. However, most children cannot conceptualize what will be true next week, much less 10 years from now. In order to get children on board, they need to be motivated. This means designing rewards that will affect them here and now. The addition of an external positive reinforcement makes a significant difference in the effectiveness of interventions for medical nonadherence (Christopherson & Mortweet, 2013; Luersen et al., 2012). Incentive plans must be clearly defined and consistently followed. Rewards must be salient to the child's specific interests. Rewards should also cost little to no money to keep them sustainable. Chapters 2 and 3 provide guidance for addressing behavioral components of treatment.

Pill Swallowing

"He won't take pills."

"I can't swallow medication."

"She chokes every time."

Despite ease in swallowing various foods throughout the day, many children experience significant difficulties when it comes to swallowing pills. We are hardwired to chew our food to protect us from choking, but our medication practices directly contradict those instincts (Osmanoglou et al., 2004). Additionally, pills vary in shape, size, and flavor, which makes it even more difficult for children to feel accustomed to swallowing medication. It's no wonder the idiom of "a hard pill to swallow" came about!

Assessing for this problem is usually straightforward. Many youth and parents alike state unequivocally that swallowing pills does not work for them. Some children refuse to take medication because they dislike the taste. Others may have a negative learning history associated with swallowing pills (e.g., choking or vomiting after taking a medication). Whatever the specific reason for pill-swallowing problems, below are some effective interventions to help youth master the act of swallowing their medication. These interventions should be performed directly with the child, with parental participation. Regardless of the age of the child, it is helpful for parents to learn the techniques and practice with the child during the visit/session. We find they benefit from seeing their child's mastery firsthand, and practicing the strategies with the parent and child together will identify any questions or barriers that could come up at home.

Interventions

When addressing medical nonadherence, we generally start with simple education. In general, providers tend to take for granted that children and their parents understand what is being asked of them. Pill swallowing is no different, and we start with a few simple steps. First, identify the different moving parts that play a role in swallowing. Instruct kids to point to their own lips, cheeks, tongue, and throat. Solicit knowledge about the function of each part. The dialogue below walks through this education with 7-year-old Gabby who was prescribed a medication that could only be taken in pill form. Use HQ Card 8.1, Learning about Swallowing (p. 195), to illustrate your description of the mechanics of swallowing.

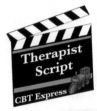

What the Therapist Can Say

THERAPIST: OK, so how do you usually swallow things?

GABBY: I put a bite in my mouth and then . . . I just swallow.

THERAPIST: Whoa!! You make it sound so easy! Did you know that swallowing is actually kind of complicated?

GABBY: Umm, no it isn't.

THERAPIST: All right, well why don't we start by breaking it down into the pieces of swallowing?

GABBY: Pieces?

THERAPIST: Yeah, what parts of your body are involved in swallowing? How about we start with your lips.

GABBY: My lips don't swallow!

THERAPIST: Haha, you're right they don't swallow, but they do get the whole thing started. What do you think these guys do to begin a swallow? (*Wiggles lips for emphasis.*)

GABBY: When you do that, you look like a horse chewing grass or something. Oh, hey, I know, lips help get the food into your mouth.

THERAPIST: That's exactly right! Now when you take your medication, I bet you put it straight into your mouth and drop it on your tongue, huh?

GABBY: Yep. I try to get it all the way so it will go down, but it never does.

THERAPIST: OK, next step is the tongue. Let me see yours!

GABBY: (*Sticks out her tongue.*)

THERAPIST: Good, you know where it is. Do you know what it does?

GABBY: It licks ice cream!

THERAPIST: Yes it does! What else does it do? How does it help you swallow?

GABBY: Hmmm. I guess it kind of pushes your food around?

THERAPIST: You got it. Your tongue pushes your food around your mouth and right to the back to push it down into your throat. Now, there are two tubes in your throat. Tell me what they do.

GABBY: They take my food to my stomach and help me breathe.

THERAPIST: Right again! The one connected to your stomach is called your esophagus. The other one is connected to your lungs and brings fresh air in through your mouth. When you eat and drink, the tube that connects to your lungs closes at the top so no food gets in where it doesn't belong.

GABBY: It closes? But then wouldn't it stop me from breathing?

THERAPIST: Nope. Let's test this out. Open your mouth like this (*opens mouth*), then take a deep breath through your nose.

GABBY: (*Takes a breath.*)

THERAPIST: See, when your mouth is busy, your nose takes over with the breathing.

GABBY: Cool.

THERAPIST: OK, so we've talked about the lips and the tongue. Now we're at the esophagus. Tell me what the esophagus does (*pointing to the esophagus on the handout*).

GABBY: You already said. It takes the food to the tummy.

THERAPIST: You're right, I gave away the answer. The esophagus is wrapped in muscles that help make sure the food makes it all the way down and into the stomach. See! That's way more complicated than you thought isn't it?

GABBY: Yeah, I guess it is.

THERAPIST: Now that we know what's happening let's get some ideas for how to make swallowing pills just as easy as swallowing ice cream!

By taking 3 brief minutes to discuss the different mechanical components of swallowing with Gabby, the therapist sets the stage to begin with interventions. In this dialogue, the therapist balances child-friendly language (e.g., *tummy*) with formal terminology (e.g., *esophagus*). This creates an interaction that is engaging and accessible to the patient, maintains credibility with parents, and introduces the patient to vocabulary that she will likely hear again from her pediatrician.

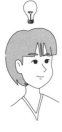

What the Therapist Can Do

Instead of lecturing the patient, the therapist makes the learning experience interactive by asking questions and responding animatedly. Gabby wasn't given the chance to tune out the therapist because she contributed just as much as the therapist did. Information delivered this way negates the need to set time aside to build rapport separately from the intervention and maximizes the efficiency of every minute of the session.

Starting Simple: How to Swallow

Ages: 4–18 years.

Module: Psychoeducation.

Purpose: Teach steps to make swallowing pills easier.

Rationale: Clear communication about the various ways to effectively swallow pills provides families with creative ideas for modifying swallowing practices to best fit each child's specific problems and preferences.

Materials: HQ Card 8.2, Take It Home: Tips for Swallowing (p. 196), and a writing utensil; cup of water.

Expected time needed: 5 minutes.

Often, pill-swallowing difficulties emerge from faulty swallowing practices. Here are some tips to help providers maximize success. Demonstrate and practice each of these steps in session to clarify exact positioning and sizes.

1. **Pill position:** *Place the pill in the middle of the tongue.*
   - Pills placed too far back on the tongue will trigger the gag reflex.
   - Pills placed right on the tip of the tongue may move around in the mouth and get stuck in the cheeks.
2. **Liquid intake:** *Make sure children are taking only a small amount of liquid to swallow with their medication.*
   - Trying to gulp down big swigs of water with pills mixed in is a great recipe for choking/gagging. Children with a history of choking or gagging may try to fix the problem by taking bigger and bigger sips of water, inadvertently making the problem worse.
   - For the right size, try asking the child to open his mouth once he's taken a sip. Sips that are too big will overflow. The best size is a sip that just fits in the child's mouth without spilling when his mouth is open.
   - One way to ensure good-sized sips is to use a straw.
   - Alternatively, a spoonful of a soft, mushy food works just as well as liquid. Consider having the child try taking pills with a bite of yogurt, applesauce, mashed potatoes, pudding, or ice cream. Place a small spoonful of the food in the center of the child's tongue and place the pill on top.
3. **Head position:** *The angle at which the child's head is tilted affects how easy it is to swallow.*
   - Children who complain that the medication gets stuck in their mouths should be taught to tilt their head gently backwards, making it easier for the tongue to push the pill directly to the esophagus.
   - Leaning the head too far back will actually make entry into the esophagus harder (try looking at the ceiling and swallowing a mouthful of saliva—not a very comfortable experience!).
   - For children who gag on medication or complain of it "getting stuck," a gentle tilt forward will help relax the esophagus and make it easier to get the medication down into the stomach.

HQ Card 8.2 gives families ideas for applying the strategies at home. This is also a good way to double-check whether the families understand the tips you are sharing. This worksheet is meant to be filled out during the visit so you can check over the responses and address any questions before the family leaves. The worksheet then serves as a visual reminder at home of the pill-swallowing tips practiced during the visit.

Sizing Up!: Graduated Practice

Ages: 4–18 years.

Module: Behavioral Experiments and Exposures.

Purpose: Teach graduated exposure to swallowing items whole.

Rationale: Completion of graduated exposures allows children to learn firsthand that they are capable of swallowing items without choking.

Materials: HQ Cards 8.3a and 8.3b, Score Card, sample and blank cards (pp. 197–198), and a writing utensil, preferred beverage, practice items (candy, fruit, etc.).

Expected time needed: 15 minutes.

Developing good swallowing techniques is just the beginning. Children need to get comfortable with swallowing something solid without chewing. The key is to start with the tiniest edibles that guarantee success. This gives children a springboard of success to motivate them to keep trying. See Figure 8.1 to get some ideas for practice items. Make sure to select things that the child *wants* to swallow. We find that an excuse to eat candy in the middle of the day helps motivate many children!

Take care to attend to allergies if providing items at your office; and remember, some of these items pose choking hazards.

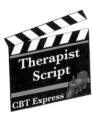

What the Therapist Can Say

"Do you like candy? What are your favorite kinds of candy? How would you like to practice swallowing some very small pieces of candy, and your reward will be even more candy? You might be thinking you are dreaming right now, but you are not. I know you have been having trouble learning to swallow your pills. So I thought we could make it more fun and easier by practicing with candy. Let me show you what I mean."

Itty bitty	Cake sprinkles (small, round, or oblong)
	Nerds candies
	Grains of rice
Tiny	Cake sprinkles (small, spherical)
Small	Mini M&M's
	Tic Tacs
	Soft fruit bits (strawberries, bananas, mango, etc.)
	Single cooked pea, corn kernel
Medium	Original M&M's
	Smarties
	Breath mint (Ice Breakers, Altoids)
	Soft fruit chunks
Large	Peanut M&M's
	Mike and Ikes
	Jelly beans
	Whole blueberry
Extra Credit	Whoppers
	Whole raspberry, blackberry
	Melon balls

FIGURE 8.1. Sizing Up!: Ideas for practice.

What the Therapist Can Do

Select one food item from each tier to plan the practices. Ideally, practices will be done in session. It is a good idea for providers to create a practice kit to keep in the office. If your clinic prohibits the provision of food to patients, work with the family to identify desired practice items to bring to their next appointment. The child should choose his or her favorite options to maximize interest and engagement.

Now the action begins! The therapist and the child (and ideally, the caregiver) will do all exercises together. Mutual practice enhances the youth's willingness to approach a feared task. Start with the smallest item. Plan to successfully swallow each item three times (i.e., one sprinkle three times) before moving on. If the child gets stuck at the next size, back up and practice the previous size again. Try picking another practice item within the same tier. For example, if a child triumphantly swallowed three mini M&M's but can't manage to swallow a regular-sized M&M, redo the practices with the mini M&M, then try swallowing some Tic Tacs. This is not a situation where we want to "push through." Repeated failures will reinforce the previous learning that swallowing pills is dangerous, uncomfortable, or impossible. Take a step back, add more victories to the child's experience, and expand the comfort zone in other ways (texture, shape) before returning to a larger item.

Be sure to celebrate victories. Each time a child successfully swallows an item, deliver specific and enthusiastic praise. Each success can be recorded on the provided Score Card (HQ Card 8.3b) to take home, which can serve as a visual reminder of the successes as well as a prompt for additional practices if needed. Therapists can use the Praise parenting block introduced in Chapter 3 to prompt parents to praise the child's efforts.

Some children only need to run through their exercises once before feeling ready to try swallowing their medication. Others may require repeated practice. Once a child consistently masters swallowing food items the same size as the required pill, he or she is ready to tackle the medication.

Youth with chronic health conditions who expect to be taking medication that may change over time might benefit from "overlearning." In these cases, youth continue practicing with items larger than their current medication. We like to call this extra credit (see Figure 8.1). By conquering practice items that exceed the size of the pills, children strengthen confidence in their ability to swallow things whole. These larger foods should be used cautiously, and the therapist should take into consideration the age of the child, the size of the medications taken, and the child's response to earlier interventions. Most children will not engage in this level of practice.

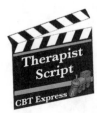

What the Therapist Can Say

In the following transcript, see how the therapist sets up this exercise with Luz, a 10-year-old girl who is having trouble swallowing her medication, and her mother. In HQ Card 8.3a, you will find her completed Score Card.

THERAPIST: Today we are going to start practicing swallowing together.

LUZ: I'm not ready! You know I can't swallow the pills!!

THERAPIST: I know that you *haven't* swallowed pills in the past! We aren't going to start out by swallowing pills. We have to start small. When you started playing violin, did you begin by playing songs?

LUZ: No. But this isn't the violin.

THERAPIST: You are right, but the way we learn anything new is usually similar. We start small! We are going to pick very small things to practice swallowing. Then, we will practice with things that are a little bit bigger, until you are an expert at swallowing. I have a box filled with lots of tiny things here that I use to help kids practice swallowing. You get to look at all the choices and pick some from each level. Then you, me, and your mom will practice swallowing them all together.

LUZ: I don't want to.

THERAPIST: OK, how about we just start by picking things from the practice box that you would be willing try to swallow. Then we can decide when to actually start swallowing them.

LUZ: That sounds OK.

THERAPIST: (*Introduces pill swallowing practice kit and gives Luz her Score Card.*) Here we have a bunch of things for you to choose from. We're going to look at all the choices for each size and you get to say one or two that you would be willing to test out. Which size do you want to pick first?

LUZ: Let's start with this one—itty bitty. Wait, these are really small.

THERAPIST: They are! We have to start with the littlest things we can find, do you know why?

LUZ: That's dumb. Of course I can swallow a sprinkle.

THERAPIST: Are you sure?

LUZ: Yes. Everyone can.

THERAPIST: Great! Then the first ones will be very easy for you. That means three easy points!

LUZ: I get points? For what?

MOTHER: I was thinking we could stop and get ice cream on the way home, if you get enough points.

LUZ: How many is enough?

THERAPIST: I'm thinking 10 points. You get one point for each time you swallow, and we will start with the sprinkles so that's three without even trying, right? How does that sound to you?

LUZ: 10 will be easy. Can I just do 10 sprinkles?

THERAPIST: Oh, I don't think that would be very helpful. It doesn't sound like you need any help learning how to swallow sprinkles! We're practicing this because it will help you when it's time to swallow your medicine.

LUZ: Fine.

THERAPIST: It sounds like you want to do sprinkles for your itty bitty level. Do you want to do chocolate or rainbow colored?

LUZ: Rainbow!!

THERAPIST: OK, pick your colors. Remember, you need three.

MOTHER: Will you pick out three colors for me too?

LUZ: OK! . . . are those Reese's Pieces?! Those are my favorite! Mom, I get to eat this now?

MOTHER: Well first you have to swallow them. Maybe you can have a couple extra so you can have some to chew too.

THERAPIST: That's a great idea. How about for each level you finish on your Score Card, you can eat three Reese's Pieces?

LUZ: Can I still get ice cream after?

MOTHER: If you earn 10 points, you can.

LUZ: I definitely can.

THERAPIST: OK, but before we get started on the practice, you have to pick something for each level. Let's get going so we can get to the good part!

The therapist outlines the exercise, provides clear expectations for Luz, and collaborates with Luz and her mother to identify incentives. The benefits of medication are never once mentioned, rather the therapist and mother highlight rewards Luz wants that she can earn immediately. Notice that the therapist does not argue with Luz or get stuck with her initial hesitation to engage in the exercise. The therapist instead focuses on what Luz is open to trying, letting her make her own decisions about whether or not to complete the exercise, giving Luz some control and keeping her engaged. A clear introduction with heavy emphasis on rewards yields strong participation in graduated exposures. In this example, ice cream is the reward, but nonfood items and activities can be used also. Therapists should work with caregivers to identify realistic rewards/activities.

Troubleshooting

"But It Tastes Sooo Gross!"

There are times when the child is struggling to swallow medication because the flavor is simply awful. No matter how skillfully you teach swallowing techniques and then practice with tasty candies, children may persist in gagging on unpleasant tasting medication.

1. Use HQ Card 8.4, Overcoming Obstacles (p. 199), with families to help them experiment with new ideas to get past this sticking point.
2. Consider talking with the physician or pharmacist about flavor options.
3. If changing the flavor is not an option, consider practicing with less appealing tasting candies for exposure to swallowing less desired tastes (flavored jelly beans are great for this type of practice since they are similar in shape to pills and come in countless flavors).

"NO!"

For flat out refusal, heels-dug-in resistance, or other noncompliant reactions to the exercises, refer to Chapter 3 on interventions for noncompliance to combine *CBT Express* strategies for a powerful punch! Use those procedures to enhance motivation and increase compliance, then come back for strategies for the pill-swallowing problems.

"I'll Choke! I Always Do!"

Children with a significant learning history of choking, gagging, or vomiting when attempting to swallow medications may be extra hesitant or fearful of doing swallowing exercises. This does not mean they cannot learn. They simply require a little extra attention to be ready to proceed with the practices.

1. Ask the child to write a list of all the things she has choked on. Next, ask the child to make a list of all the things she is able to swallow without choking.
2. Increase the value of and/or frequency of rewards to be earned. For example, instead of getting a prize for passing each level on the Score Card, a child would earn a prize for every swallow.

HQ Card 8.4 will help you guide families through problem-solving the barriers they have encountered.

Adherence to a Medication Regimen

"We forget."

"We decided we didn't want to go that route."

"I hate the way it makes me feel."

"It wasn't working so we stopped."

Adherence to a medication regimen is defined in this chapter as consuming the medication at the dose and frequency prescribed by the provider. The bulk of our discussion will address underuse of medication, the most common referral question. Overuse of medication is typically indicative of substance abuse, which falls outside the scope of this chapter. For therapists who work in primary care or multidisciplinary settings, conducting team appointments with the prescribing providers when targeting medication regimen allows for seamless integration of accurate medical information and behavioral health interventions.

Indications of nonadherence to a medication regimen can include parents openly expressing complaints or confusion about medication, absence of or infrequent refill requests and lab results that show negligible levels of the medication in the body. More subtle signs may include families complaining of persistent side effects. For many medications, side effects emerge early but fade over time. If a child is taking the medication inconsistently, his or her body does not have the opportunity to acclimate and unpleasant side effects may linger.

(Note: This may also be a sign that the patient is taking more than the prescribed dose, though it could also be a side effect occurring in the context of adherence to the medical regimen. These side effects should always be discussed with the physician.) Similarly, families may deny symptom relief despite the prescribing provider's expectations (Wu et al., 2013).

Interventions

Regardless of whether there is a clear problem, it is always a good idea to assess a family's understanding and execution of the regimen. HQ Card 8.5, Fast Facts for My Medications, can be completed before the appointment while the family is in the waiting room or completed quickly with the family at the start of the visit. HQ Card 8.5 gathers information about basic understanding as well as actual implementation of the regimen and highlights areas for intervention. In addition, the Fast Facts HQ Card can be used with families to provide introductory psychoeducation when new prescriptions are given to help set up strategies for successfully following the regimen.

Fast Facts

Ages: 0–18 years (completed by caregivers for children under 8 years).

Module: Psychoeducation.

Purpose: Gather information about the family's understanding of the prescribed regimen.

Rationale: The data the family provides on the HQ Card give a clear framework for treatment targets, whether it is fundamental misunderstanding about the medication regimen or barriers to the execution of the regimen.

Materials: HQ Cards 8.5a and 8.5b, Fast Facts for My Medications, sample and blank cards (pp. 200–201), and a writing utensil.

Expected time needed: 15 minutes.

HQ Card 8.5b can be given to the family to complete in the waiting room or can be completed together with the therapist. Drawing from the information provided in HQ Card 8.5b, you can quickly identify where the family is missing important information. Brief, targeted psychoeducation easily addresses these roadblocks.

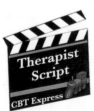

What the Therapist Can Say

"I know there are a lot of details to keep track of with your child's treatment. This worksheet includes some areas that many families tell us can be hard to recall about their child's medication regimen. I thought we could take a look at it together and see if there are areas I may be able to help simplify or clarify with you."

What the Therapist Can Do

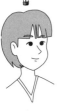

Review the necessary timing for medication doses and provide concrete examples. Instead of just saying "in the morning," use details like "before you leave for school" or "with breakfast." Also clarify how the child should be taking the medication. Does it matter if the child eats immediately before or after taking the medication? Can the family cut up or crush the pill to facilitate consumption? Addressing these questions from the start can help avoid unintentional interference with the effectiveness of the medication.

Anticipate barriers the family may encounter and preemptively problem-solve. Specify how much food is needed with each dose (e.g., a couple bites of a banana, a full meal). Give a "window of opportunity." If a medication should be taken in the morning and is forgotten, how late in the day can the dose be taken? Discuss what to do if the family runs out of medication before refilling. Interventions to minimize such problems are outlined in the next section. Arming families with this information clarifies expectations and enhances compliance. Make sure to add any of these details to the HQ Card.

Explicitly address motivation when talking about medication with families. While parents need to understand the short- and long-term outcomes expected with both compliance and noncompliance, children deal in the concrete and the immediate. Explanations of how this medication will benefit them in the future sound like mildly annoying white noise. Directly connect compliance to their personal goals: "If you do not take this medication, you cannot get your driver's license." If medication does not impact the child's preferred activities, implement an incentive plan (see introduction to this chapter).

To review: Once you've addressed the identified targets from HQ Card 8.5, give the family a new HQ Card and ask them to fill it in using the information discussed in the appointment. This provides the family with a concrete (and correct) guide they can take home, as well as giving you another opportunity to assess their understanding. Some families may find it helpful to take a picture of the completed worksheet with their phone so they have a handy summary of their medication plan. HQ Card 8.5a is a sample filled out with 12-year-old Alex's family.

Piece It Together

Ages: 0–18 years (completed by caregivers for children under 8 years).

Modules: Target Monitoring; Basic Behavioral Tasks.

Purpose: Identify ways to help the family comply with the medication regimen.

Rationale: Creating a clear routine for medication doses eliminates confusion and enhances compliance, especially when supplemented with helpful reminders.

Materials: HQ Card 8.6, Piece It Together (p. 202), and a writing utensil; mobile device (optional).

Expected time needed: 5 minutes for the worksheet alone, 15 minutes when setting alarms, downloading apps, and practicing.

For families who communicate a clear understanding of the function of the medication and the prescribed regimen, but struggle to remember to take the doses, use HQ Card 8.6 to brainstorm ways to make it easier to stay on top of the medication routine.

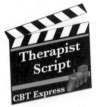

What the Therapist Can Say

"Like many families, your schedule is very busy. You have work responsibilities, your online class, helping the kids with homework, and the day-to-day chores and tasks that seem never-ending. It is not surprising that medication sometimes gets forgotten in the midst of your busy lives. I wonder if it would be helpful to brainstorm together some strategies that may help your family stay on top of the medication schedule. I could also share some ideas that other families like your family have found helpful."

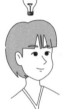

What the Therapist Can Do

Therapists can use the strategies below to design the most impactful interventions for each individual patient. Brainstorming and talking through options with the family helps make sure the plan is realistic and increases the likelihood of adherence to the plan.

Storage

Keep medication easily accessible for administration times. Store medications where they are taken (e.g., morning doses can be kept in the kitchen) and where they may be needed (e.g., rescue inhaler kept in Mom's purse). (Note: Consult with the prescribing provider to determine what, if any, is a safe amount of medication that can be stored with less restricted access.)

Supervision

Assign roles for who will retrieve the medication and supervise the administration. Often families take a "whoever is around" approach to medication monitoring. This practice can lead to "I thought you did it" situations. Identifying the responsible party keeps expectations clear and makes it harder for medication doses to slip through the cracks.

Tracking

Maintain records. This delivers immediate feedback to families about their adherence. Provide a simple worksheet such as HQ Card 8.7, My Medicine Monitor (p. 203), that patients can use to track when they take medications. Offer sheets of stickers to younger children to use to mark off doses. Being creative helps to engage youth in the regimen! Ask families to then bring their records to appointments to easily show providers adherence. When youth present to appointments with record forms, shower them with praise and enthusiasm for their accomplishments! See "Take Advantage of Technology" for electronic tracking ideas.

Reminders

Busy families need extra boosts to remember. Work with families to create reminders and ask families where they can post the signs in their home to help out. Our favorites are by doors, next to light switches, and on mirrors.

Take Advantage of Technology

Take advantage of mobile devices already integrated into a family's everyday life. Capitalize on alarm functions in cellphones, personal tablets, wristwatches, and fitness monitors (e.g., Fitbit). Set alarms on devices in session. Have fun picking ring tones and assigning labels to the alarms! This ensures the family sets up the alarm effectively to notify the people who will be responsible for medication dose times at the right time, and on the correct days. If a caregiver works nights, setting the alarms on her phone probably will not augment compliance for an evening medication. For those times that only one parent attends a visit but the other parent will be in charge of medication, have the parent who is present set an alarm for the next time both parents will be together so that they remember to coordinate alarms and other reminders on their phones in accordance with the plan.

There are also a number of mobile applications that families may download to smartphones or tablets to help monitor adherence (see "Resources" on p. 186). Download and set up mobile apps while in session. Practice logging a dose and set the reminders. Make sure all family members understand how to use the app and how to review the data that is logged. This gives families another opportunity to show providers their understanding of the medication regimen.

Helping or Harming?

Ages: Any parent/caregiver.

Module: Target Monitoring; Cognitive Restructuring.

Purpose: Identify thoughts about medication that interfere with regimen adherence.

Rationale: Learning a family's fears, doubts, or unreasonable expectations paves the way to creating more balanced and reasonable perceptions and can increase adherence.

Materials: HQ Cards 8.8a and 8.8b, Helping or Harming?, sample and blank cards (pp. 204–205), and a writing utensil.

Expected time needed: 5 minutes.

Some parents harbor ambivalence about medication, which typically translates to intermittent adherence. Ascertain whether distorted cognitions are present by asking parents to share their thoughts on medication. Parents may be hesitant to express concerns and simply nod in agreement when a physician outlines prescriptions. Explicitly solicit parents' thoughts about medication, including expectations, concerns, and doubts.

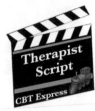

What the Therapist Can Say

"Sometimes parents have concerns or worries about their child's medication and they hesitate to bring them up because they just want to do what is right for their child. What are the questions or concerns that go through your mind when you think about your child's diagnosis and medications?"

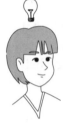

What the Therapist Can Do

When caregivers have unidentified or unexpressed negative thoughts about a medication or the illness requiring the medication, they may be less likely to adhere to the regimen. By including parents or other caregivers in your work on medical adherence, you can help identify thoughts and beliefs related to the illness and treatment, and then work with the families on any distortions or misperceptions that may be getting in the way.

The dialogue below illustrates how a therapist used this technique to uncover a mother's discomfort with the stool softener her 5-year-old son, Ben, was prescribed to treat constipation. The dialogue below picks up while the therapist is reviewing HQ Card 8.8 with Ben's mother.

THERAPIST: I see you didn't do much shading here.

MOM: Not really, no.

THERAPIST: Then right here you wrote down a big zero under the best possible outcome and "diarrhea and accidents" under worst possible outcomes.

MOM: Yeah.

THERAPIST: Tell me what's been getting in the way.

MOM: It's just that I know the doctor said the medication will help him, but I've taken a similar medication before and I had a really hard time with it. It gave me terrible gas and I was running to the bathroom all the time. I just don't see how that's much better than being constipated.

THERAPIST: That makes sense. It sounds like you think this medication has a good chance of causing more problems than there already are.

MOM: Mm-hmm.

THERAPIST: No wonder you're having a hard time giving him the medication the way the doctor prescribed it! Do you think the pediatrician would have filled this form out differently than you did?

MOM: Yeah, I mean if we filled it out based on how the medication was explained to us, I guess the best possible outcome would say no more constipation.

THERAPIST: And if the medication works like the pediatrician said it would, there would be other benefits too?

MOM: Well, if he's not constipated he won't have accidents as often, and it shouldn't hurt when he goes to the bathroom.

THERAPIST: That sounds consistent with what the pediatrician said. Have you guys tested out the medication at all?

MOM: Not really. I gave it to him for a week or two after our appointment last month and it didn't do anything. That's why I left a big part of the pill unshaded on that sheet. Since it didn't seem to help, I didn't want to give him too much and have things get worse. I know the dose is different for this medication than what I was taking, so I don't really think it's going to be bad for him. It just didn't really seem like it was doing anything, so why keep taking it?

THERAPIST: Got it. So mostly you don't think this medication will do much for Ben, but if it does have an effect, the chances are it wouldn't be helpful.

Using HQ Card 8.8 as a platform for discussion, the therapist identified Ben's mother's doubts about the medication's efficacy as well as her concerns about the medication. Now that the therapist has a clear understanding of the beliefs that are interfering with the successful execution of the medication regimen, the therapist can intervene on the misperception using one of the interventions below.

Test It Out

Ages: Children ages 12–18 years and parents/caregivers.

Module: Cognitive Restructuring.

Purpose: Test out distorted beliefs about medication.

Rationale: Gathering evidence about beliefs, just like detectives follow clues, helps patients to "solve the case" regarding their perceptions of medication.

Materials: HQ Card 8.9, Test It Out (p. 206), and a writing utensil.

Expected time needed: 10 minutes.

Once the distorted perception is identified, work with the family to gather evidence that supports or refutes that conclusion. Using Ben's mother's thoughts from the example above, she stated "nothing changed" when she administered the medication. Below the therapist works with the mother on this thought.

What the Therapist Can Say

THERAPIST: OK, so thinking back to those 2 weeks when you did test out the medication—did Ben take it every day?

MOM: Yes, I gave him the pill an hour before bedtime, like the doctor suggested.

THERAPIST: Great! Now the last time you were here, Ben had been having bowel movements once or twice a week, with accidents happening daily.

MOM: Yes, and he was having tummy aches all the time too. Just like he is now.

THERAPIST: Tummy aches, accidents, and infrequent poops, got it. When he was taking the medication, how often did he have accidents?

MOM: I'm not sure.

BEN: I got a prize! At school!

THERAPIST: A prize?

MOM: Oh that's right. His teacher gives him rewards for having accident-free days. He earned a prize for having 3 days with no accidents.

BEN: And then I got to eat lunch with Mrs. Appel!

THERAPIST: That sounds so fun! That was for no accidents?

MOM: Yeah, he earned two prizes in a row, I think, so she wanted to do something extra special.

THERAPIST: Wow!! Good for you, Ben! It sounds like right around the time you guys began the medication there were at least a few days without accidents.

MOM: That's true. He also was going to the bathroom a lot.

THERAPIST: You mean many times a day?

MOM: No, he was pooping more. Almost every day. I remember because he kept asking for help with wiping.

BEN: I didn't want to get all messy.

MOM: I forgot what a poop machine you were that week!

THERAPIST: OK, so it sounds like the medication may have been working some after all.

MOM: Yes, but he was still having accidents at home.

THERAPIST: Were they happening every day?

MOM: No. There were a few on the weekend. His sister had a soccer tournament that weekend. We had to change pants twice on both days.

THERAPIST: Uh-oh, that definitely sounds like a hard time. Do you remember if he was having accidents on other days?

MOM: Not really, no. I just remember after that weekend I was so fed up with the accidents, the medication seemed like it either wasn't helping or it was making the diarrhea worse so we stopped. I think he was fine for like a day or so, but then he almost immediately went back to the daily accidents.

THERAPIST: It sounds like the medication may have started to get Ben on a more regular bathroom schedule at first.

MOM: Yeah, he did win those prizes at school. I forgot about that. Maybe it was helping at first.

THERAPIST: Was there anything else that may have contributed to the accidents at the soccer fields?

MOM: I mean we had to hike to get to the bathrooms. He told us he needed to go. We just never made it in time.

THERAPIST: If he had quick access to the bathroom do you think that might've made a difference?

MOM: I guess it's possible. But I gave him the medication a handful of other days after that and it definitely did not make a difference. Other than those 2 weeks, the accidents have been the same.

THERAPIST: You tried it again, giving it every night?

MOM: No, just when I thought about it, or when I was really frustrated about cleaning up yet another accident.

THERAPIST: OK, so then we have some good evidence that just taking it sometimes doesn't seem to work. It also looks like we have some good evidence that taking it every night at the same time was starting to improve things. What are your thoughts about trying it daily again to see if the benefits increase over time?

By asking questions about frequency of bowel movements and accidents, the therapist helped Ben's mother to evaluate her beliefs regarding the medication's ineffectiveness. In the first weeks when Ben had been taking the medication as prescribed, Ben and his mother each identified evidence that the medication was helping. When circumstances arose that posed challenges for the family, it was easy to draw the conclusion that the medication was ineffective. Ben stopped taking his medication regularly and the daily accidents returned.

What the Therapist Can Do

On HQ Card 8.9, the therapist works with Ben's mother to fill in evidence for and against the medication's effectiveness. This information can then be used to identify how and when the medication has the strongest effects, as well as what things interfere with the effectiveness of the medication regimen. The final step is to have the parent decide whether he or she is willing to give the medication a try.

This exercise can also be completed with adolescent patients, testing their own beliefs about prescribed medications. Instead of gathering and then testing the caregiver's thoughts as was done above with Ben's mother, the procedure is completed directly with the patient.

Older youth often prefer to manage their own medication. The assertion of independence is developmentally typical of teens, however many of these youth need support to maintain compliance. Give teens choices to honor autonomous decision making while also providing structure. Present yourself as part of a teen's team, not as an authority demanding compliance. Clearly define consequences of continued nonadherence.

What the Therapist Can Say

In this exchange, the therapist works with 14-year-old Raylon to devise a plan to improve her compliance with her medication regimen.

THERAPIST: We need to figure out how to make it easier for you to remember to take your medication.

RAYLON: I don't need help. I'll just do it now. I get that it's important.

THERAPIST: I know you understand. It's not that I think you suck at this. You've got a lot going on right now. I want to work with you to figure out how to make this as easy as possible so it doesn't have to be another thing for you to worry about. We've got to recruit some people to play on your team. You can't win a ball game alone.

RAYLON: Well, if my mom tells me I have to take my medication it just makes me angry that she's treating me like a baby, so sometimes I just don't take it to piss her off.

THERAPIST: Is there anyone else besides your mom who could help us so that you two don't have to fight about the medication anymore?

RAYLON: Not really. I mean, my sister is around sometimes, but she's just as annoying, acting like she's my second mother or something.

THERAPIST: OK, so you are open to building a team to help, but everyone who could be on your team is not allowed?

RAYLON: Haha, I guess so. See, that's why I'll just do it myself.

THERAPIST: How about we come up with a way that your mom can help double-check without being annoying?

RAYLON: Like what?

THERAPIST: Hmmm—is there a way we could ask your mom to check that wouldn't make you mad?

RAYLON: She won't do it. No matter what I say to her, she always comes at me like, "Did you forget to take your medication?!" She just assumes I'm messing up.

THERAPIST: So what would be a better way to ask? A way that wouldn't feel like she's accusing you?

RAYLON: Could I just tell her every time I take it? Or text. Texting would be way better.

THERAPIST: I think you are on to something. Texting could really cut down on the arguing. So what happens if you take it but you forget to text her? We need a way for her to be the one checking in so you have a backup reminder.

RAYLON: All right, fine. How about if she texts me the medication emoji?

THERAPIST: That sounds reasonable. What time do you think is appropriate to give you enough of a chance to remember on your own before she sends you the reminder?

RAYLON: Um . . . I'm supposed to take it at night, so I guess 10 would be good. That's right when I'm getting ready for bed usually.

THERAPIST: And how will Mom know if you took the medication?

RAYLON: I will text back the thumbs up emoji.

THERAPIST: Great. And how many misses do you think you should get before we give Mom a promotion and make her the supreme medication boss?

RAYLON: Arggggh. I mean, I guess it's three strikes, right? That's usually the rule.

THERAPIST: OK, so to be clear—you are in charge of your medication. After you take it, you text your mom to let her know you did it. If you don't text by 10:00 P.M., she'll text you a medicine emoji to remind you. If you miss three doses *total* before our next appointment, your mom is in charge of your medication every day.

The therapist and Raylon work together to outline reasonable parameters that support compliance in developmentally appropriate ways. As the therapist works with Raylon to identify ways to increase support, Raylon continues to point out all the reasons why she doesn't need help and why she can just handle the medication on her own. Instead of arguing with her or pointing out her past failure to do so, the therapist provides suggestions for how Raylon can move forward. Without demanding Raylon follow strict guidelines, the therapist sets up clear expectations for Raylon and her mother, and prompts Raylon to set her own limits. By respecting her drive for autonomy, the therapist engages Raylon in making the plans, likely enhancing her willingness to follow them.

Troubleshooting

"We Never Remember to Get Refills Until We're All Out."

In addition to tracking daily medication administration, parents need to keep an eye on refills. Problem-solve how to keep from running out of medication.

1. Set calendar reminders for refills 5 days before the current prescription runs out.
2. Sign up for auto refills if offered by the pharmacy or insurance provider.
3. Contact the insurance company to enroll in prescriptions delivered by mail.

"This Medication Is Expensive."

For some families, the cost of certain medications may be prohibitive. Although this is a major barrier to adherence, many families are hesitant to bring it up with providers.

1. Ask about how the cost of medication is affecting the family.
2. Investigate whether there are coupons or discount cards the family can use.
3. Consult with the prescribing provider about alternatives that will be less costly (and thus easier to maintain).

"It's Too Hard to Take the Medication This Way."

When families with a good plan continue to struggle with adherence, they may be failing at the actual consumption of the medication.

1. For problems with swallowing pills, see *CBT Express* interventions earlier in this chapter.
2. For parenteral, or non-oral, administration, consult with the prescribing provider about alternatives. Identify particular difficulties associated with route of delivery and help parents problem-solve how to overcome the barrier.

"Nope—Not Taking It."

If a child is not interested in complying with the medication prescription, adherence becomes impossible.

1. Review the incentive plan the family is using. Check that rewards are motivating for the patient and being delivered consistently.
2. See Chapter 3 on noncompliance for more ideas about how to address defiant behaviors.

If a parent's negative beliefs about the prescribed medication are unyielding, it may be time to explore alternatives.

1. Collaborate with the prescribing provider to determine if there is another class of medication that the parents may be more willing to try out.
2. Investigate other evidence-based treatments. For many conditions, medication may be the most effective treatment, but there may be other helpful options that are less potent. For example, stimulant medication shows the best effect on ADHD, but there are various nonstimulant options that demonstrate an (albeit lesser) effect.

Resources

Free printable calendars: *www.calendarlabs.com*

Apps that can be used to track daily activities (e.g., medication doses): HabitBull, Productive, GoalTracker

Medication-specific apps, especially useful for complex medication regimens: Mango Health, Medisafe Medication Reminder, CareZone

Adherence to a Nutrition Plan

"I can't get him to stop eating chips."

"She doesn't like vegetables."

"She keeps sneaking food."

"This food is disgusting!"

"It just doesn't seem like enough food."

"But everyone else drinks soda!"

Nutrition plans are prescribed for a variety of reasons: obesity, disordered eating, allergies, chronic medical conditions (e.g., diabetes), failure to thrive, and more. Nonadherence to the nutrition plan is evident by failure to gain/lose weight, persisting negative outcomes related to chronic medical conditions, and repeated visits to urgent care/the emergency department.

Nutrition plans require major household changes, altering the way families shop for, store, cook, and serve food. The added burden of transforming eating habits may seem impossible for families with working parents, multiple children, and/or a child with a chronic medical condition. Just as with medication regimens, parents must understand how a nutrition plan will help their child. It is helpful for parents to understand short-term and long-term outcomes of nonadherence.

Interventions

Compliance with a nutrition plan often requires substantial efforts with little immediate reward (e.g., it may take several weeks on a nutrition plan for obesity before weight loss occurs). Families are grateful for clear guidelines regarding expectations. Help orient them to find signs of progress instead of waiting for major outcomes.

Color Your Food Choices: Green, Yellow, Red!

Ages: 5–18 years.

Module: Psychoeducation.

Purpose: Provide a broad outline of the nutrition plan to help the family understand which foods can be eaten regularly, which should be eaten sparingly, and which to restrict or remove from the child's diet.

Rationale: Giving the family a framework in which to understand the guiding principles of the nutrition plan will increase adherence to the plan.

Materials: HQ Card 8.10, Green, Yellow, Red (p. 207), and a writing utensil.

Expected time needed: 5 minutes.

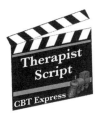

What the Therapist Can Say

"You mentioned it was hard to know what you are allowed to eat and it seems like there are no 'good' foods allowed anymore. I have this paper here that can quickly help you identify what foods are 'in the green,' meaning they are good for you to eat. We can also talk about which foods are in the red and should be avoided but may be OK for a once-a-week treat if you eat green at other times. Would you rather we write the names of the foods on the worksheet, or draw or cut-out pictures of the foods?"

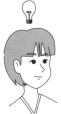

What the Therapist Can Do

Use HQ Card 8.10 to clarify the nutrition plan. Specify what foods are desired and what foods should be avoided. Green, Yellow, Red sets up the guidelines for the nutrition plan. For example, "green" foods for a child struggling with obesity could be "green vegetables," while "red" foods could include "soda pop" or "potato chips." Once the family expresses understanding of the framework, collaborate on the My Shopping

List activity by generating specific examples of foods the family is willing to buy and has access to (e.g., zucchini and green beans) and specific items the child historically has eaten but must now work to deliberately avoid (e.g., soda and potato chips). Families can complete this exercise by writing in ideas, drawing images, or pasting pictures into the columns. Review portion sizes with concrete examples; for example, one serving of vegetables should be about the size of your fist.

My Shopping List

Ages: 5–18 years.

Module: Psychoeducation.

Purpose: Identify specific foods to eat more of and foods to avoid.

Rationale: Create a clear and specific list to give the family a concrete guide to use when grocery shopping.

Materials: HQ Card 8.11, My Shopping List (p. 208), drawing/writing utensils, camera (optional, can be on cellphone), printed or digital images of desired versus avoided foods (optional).

Expected time needed: 5 minutes.

Once families understand which foods to stay away from and which foods to increase access to, they can build a grocery shopping list to take to the store. HQ Card 8.11 and the My Shopping List intervention can be started during a brief interaction with the family. Then this *CBT Express* intervention can be taken home to continue to build a clear plan for successful food shopping and meal planning.

What the Therapist Can Do

Have the family start to fill out HQ Card 8.11 during the visit and provide feedback on their food selections. Facilitate communication and family problem solving. Encourage families to select one "treat" to buy each trip to allow them some access to favorite items. Doing so can reduce the likelihood of bingeing and improves compliance with the nutrition plan as a whole.

The best way to enhance a child's compliance with the prescribed nutrition plan is to eliminate undesired foods from the household. Depending on the stringency of the plan, this may not be possible. In those cases, work with parents to design a storage plan where "bad" foods are hard to find and "good" foods are readily available. Keep unwanted foods on high shelves, in locked cabinets, or other difficult to access places (e.g., parents' bedroom, in the garage, or in the trunk of a car). Create a snack basket that sits on the kitchen counter or in the fridge and contains several options that fit within the nutrition plan.

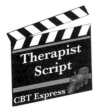

What the Therapist Can Say

"Most children like junk food because it's tasty and it's ready. We can't affect how delicious potato chips are, but we can make it much easier to pick a piece of fruit or a yogurt for a snack by keeping them clearly identified and in easy reach. What foods from the nutrition plan do you think would be most appealing to your child?"

Scavenger Hunt

Ages: 3–18 years.

Module: Basic Behavioral Tasks.

Purpose: Locate where to find desired foods and where to move (or remove) undesired foods.

Rationale: Specifying locations encourages the family to imagine how the nutrition plan fits in their home, transforming the plan from theoretical to realistic.

Materials: HQ Card 8.12, Scavenger Hunt (p. 209), (or blank paper), drawing/writing utensils.

Expected time needed: 10 minutes.

HQ Card 8.12 is designed to help families figure out how they will restructure their homes to facilitate adherence to the nutrition plan. It is a fun and engaging way to get families thinking about where food is or should be kept for optimal success with the plan. It also provides opportunities to personalize the plan for the family.

What the Therapist Can Do

Using HQ Card 8.12, ask the child to provide snack ideas and list where the snacks can be found in the family kitchen. Alternatively, a child may opt to draw his or her family's specific kitchen layout, then add the locations of approved snacks.

Another alternative is to create a visual list of options for meals and snacks. Lists can be made with pictures, drawings, cut-out labels, or words depending on the family's preferences. Families may choose to create their own menu or fill in HQ Card 8.13, Family Menu.

Mario was struggling to make healthy breakfast choices when he and his father were seen for a follow-up clinic visit. The therapist introduced HQ Card 8.13, and Mario and his father worked together to implement a visual plan that also allowed Mario some independence in selecting snacks. Mario was prescribed a gluten-free diet. His provider had previously identified breakfast options to replace his go-to pastries. Mario selected three favorites from the list, then used his father's phone to take pictures of his choices. His father later printed the pictures and put them on the fridge so that Mario could pick from his menu each morning instead of arguing with his father about what was available.

The Family Menu

Ages: 4–18 years.

Module: Basic Behavioral Tasks.

Purpose: Give the family a specific guide to meals that meets requirements of the nutrition plan.

Rationale: Instead of only providing sample foods, a menu illustrates for the family that adherence to the nutrition plan is attainable, while simultaneously creating a visual reminder of how to follow the plan.

Materials: HQ Card 8.13, The Family Menu (p. 210), drawing/writing utensils, camera/pictures (optional).

Expected time needed: 10 minutes.

Some families benefit from or even ask for more specific guidelines for meals. For these families, helping them create a Family Menu can reduce stress and arguing about meals, lessen nightly decisions about what to make for dinner, and prevent sibling spats if different foods are available to siblings. This was the case with Gracie, whose mom wanted to follow the nutritional recommendations but was overwhelmed with the constant monitoring and decision making about food.

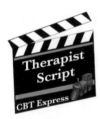

What the Therapist Can Say

"You mentioned that the nightly meal planning is wearing on you, and you worry that Gracie isn't getting what she should nutritionally. That sounds like it is really stressing you out. Some families find it easier to set a menu for a week at a time. This reduces the daily decisions about food, and actually helps you plan for trips to the grocery store. It can also help avoid the arguments between Gracie and her brother, since she is getting jealous if he is eating something she isn't supposed to have."

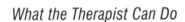

What the Therapist Can Do

Encourage families to eat meals together. Caregivers can monitor meal portions and directly control food choices. Whenever possible, include at least one dish per meal that the whole family can eat. Children are likely to feel less stigmatized by their nutrition plan when they share food with the family.

Make sure meals are fun. Brainstorm games to be played during meals to keep table time fun. Many families enjoy Best and Worst, where each family member shares the best part of his or her day and the worst part. The Alphabet Game includes family members taking turns picking a topic, then going around the table saying one thing that fits the theme that starts with each letter of the alphabet (e.g., Cereals—Apple Jacks, Bran, Cheerios). Family meals are also enjoyable for children, as they present opportunities to delight in their parents' attention. For parents with alternative work schedules, divide meals into "kids' mealtime" and "parents' mealtime," and encourage one parent to sit with the kids as they eat to maintain supervision as well as positive reinforcement.

It can be harder to adhere to a nutrition plan when parents share the same health concerns. For example, youth with obese parents are up to 12 times more likely to become obese (Fuemmeler, Lovelady, Zucker, & Ostbyte, 2013). Parents may not be interested in or ready to make changes to their own behavior patterns.

Cultural Considerations

Food is inextricably intermingled with cultural values. Hearing providers explain that favored or commonplace cultural foods are now off limits due to their health implications often feels insensitive or unrealistic to families. In some cultures, food is representative of parents' fundamental ability to nurture their child; thus, directing families to limit serving size during meals is akin to instructing them to fail as parents. Ideal body size and shape also vary between cultures, making discussions about weight fraught with misunderstandings.

The critical component to navigating the discrepancies between cultural norms and nutrition plan prescriptions is understanding. Take extra time to learn about traditional dishes and the significance of food for the family. Be sure to explain very clearly the rationale for the nutrition plan, anchoring the discussion with concrete health-related symptoms that the plan aims to address. Emphasize in your discussions that it is not the cultural values that are a problem, but the _____ (uncontrolled blood sugar, gastrointestinal distress, or obesity that limits the child from participating in gym class, etc.). Prepare yourself to engage in transparent, nondefensive, and validating discussions with parents who very likely experience discrimination regularly. Engage families in brainstorming alternative foods that are in line with the nutrition plan *and* the family's culture.

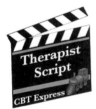

What the Therapist Can Say

In the following example, the therapist is working with a Mexican family whose 6-year-old son, Cesar, was prescribed a nutrition plan due to prediabetic symptoms.

DAD: We know Cesar is a little overweight, but he is a hungry boy. He is growing. You cannot expect us to stop feeding him. And the doctor told us that he cannot eat tortillas or rice anymore. The doctor said that what we are feeding him is hurting him. That is not right. We have traditions and you cannot possibly expect us to just give up our culture because we moved the United States.

THERAPIST: You are absolutely right, we do not expect you to turn away from your heritage to help Cesar get healthy.

DAD: What do you mean "healthy"? He isn't sick. There is nothing wrong with him. Just because he doesn't look like the other children doesn't mean we are doing something wrong.

THERAPIST: I completely agree. And I don't think you are doing something wrong. Cesar's pediatrician explained to us that Cesar is showing some symptoms inside of his body that are worrisome. The pediatrician is not concerned about how Cesar looks, but rather how healthy his body is.

DAD: Then why did the pediatrician talk about his weight?

THERAPIST: The pediatrician is trying to help Cesar's body be healthier. One very important way to do that is to reduce his weight.

DAD: But look at us, we are a big family. Both his mother and I are overweight, but we do not have any problems.

THERAPIST: That's great that you are both healthy. Right now, Cesar is showing some serious signs in his blood that he may develop diabetes soon if we don't work together to help him. Diabetes is a lifelong disease that will make Cesar's life much harder if we can't make some changes for him.

DAD: How is giving up our traditions going to help him?

THERAPIST: Let's look at ways we can make little changes to how Cesar is eating to help his body. We want to look at two parts—what is he eating and how much is he eating. We want this plan to be realistic so that you can do it at home.

Throughout this exchange, the therapist maintains the focus on Cesar's health as indicated by the symptoms he is experiencing rather than arguing with the family about whether the cultural values are under attack.

Families with limited resources often note that they have neither the time nor the money to buy and prepare food that fits within the meal plan. Ready-to-eat meals are quick and typically inexpensive. To address these concerns, it is helpful to provide families with information about how they can logistically adhere to the meal plan. Quick and healthy recipes are readily available from an internet search. Select a handful of recipes that seem to fit with the needs of the families with whom you are working and print them out. It is also a great idea to post seasonal lists of fruits and vegetables in your office or waiting room to give families ideas about what produce is currently available at a lower cost. Also, be sure to give families HQ Card 8.14, Money-Saving Tips for Healthy Eating (p. 211), when reviewing the nutrition plan. However, keep in mind the family's specific needs and resources and modify the list as appropriate.

Keeping a Balance Sheet

Ages: 8–18 years and parents.

Module: Cognitive Restructuring.

Purpose: Generate a balanced perspective that includes both upsides and downsides to adhering to the nutrition plan.

Rationale: Encouraging patients and their families to consider all aspects of the nutrition plan helps to unstick helpless or resentful perceptions and promote willingness to try out new behavior patterns.

Materials: HQ Cards 8.15a, 8.15b, and 8.15c, Pros and Cons, sample and blank cards (pp. 212–214), and a writing utensil.

Expected time needed: 10 minutes.

Parents and children alike often feel resentful about needing to modify their eating habits. Children begrudge the mandate to give up favored foods and follow different rules than siblings or peers. Parents object to making changes to their own diets when it's not their medical condition that needs to be treated. Working with children and parents to make their own Pros and Cons list helps shift perspectives and makes the rewards more notable.

What the Therapist Can Do

Begin the exercise by having the patient and parent mark their level of interest in making the changes recommended by the meal plan along the line at the top. Next, ask the patient and parent(s) to write down two to three benefits and two to three disadvantages to following the nutrition plan. HQ Cards 8.15a and 8.15b show Jaimie and her mother's completed lists and ratings.

While it is helpful to point out advantages that you might note, if the child or parent doesn't agree, adding your ideas to the list will not help shift the family's thinking. For example, in HQ Card 8.15a, encouraging Jaimie to add "getting to try new things" to her pros list probably isn't going to help her because she doesn't *want* to have to try new foods.

Once the list is written, work with the family to adjust overgeneralizations and catastrophic conclusions. Be sure to be balanced in your review of the lists. The cons associated with a nutrition plan really are tough for families. By empathizing with the family about the cons, you earn credibility needed to review the pros. After you've discussed both sides of the list, ask the family to rerate their interest in making changes.

Troubleshooting

"It Doesn't Matter What I Pack for Lunch; He's Always Eating Pizza at the Cafeteria."

The older the child is, the harder it is to control food choices. Parents may feel like they have no hope of impacting the child's food intake.

1. Help parents loosen all-or-nothing thinking. Try asking the family to write out everything the child ate yesterday, then point out opportunities for the parents to have had some impact.
2. Plan for breaks: A rigid diet may create a sense of hopelessness or fatigue in parents or the child. Allot the child one or two treats a week to give some room for indulgence. (Be sure to confirm with the nutritionist or physician that a treat would be safe to recommend, or get guidance about appropriate treats to offer.)

"I Want Nuggets. I'm Not Eating That."

No matter the age of the child, parents learn quickly that children cannot be forced to eat.

1. For children who are defiant at mealtimes and refuse to eat, instruct parents to offer choices: "You can eat this meal or not. This food will be ready for you when you are hungry."
2. Help parents decide how to set limits on this. Is there a deadline for when the meal must be eaten, or can the child decide to return to the meal at bedtime?
3. It is critical that parents understand that allowing children to eat alternate foods reinforces the children for refusing meals, and thus they are far less likely to ever be compliant. Let's be honest, how many children willingly cut out their favorite foods?
4. Refusing food produces quick natural consequences that are hard to ignore. Even the most strong-willed child will only go to bed hungry a few nights before realizing there is only one way to get fed. (Note: This intervention is not appropriate for youth prescribed a nutrition plan to gain weight.)

"Ewwww!!!"

Some children are hesitant to try new foods. This can significantly interfere with nutrition plans for children who must make substantial changes to eating habits.

1. Introduce new foods with a "three-strikes" rule. Children must try one bite of a new food three times before issuing a verdict.
2. Youth with highly restrictive palates may require a more graduated approach. In these situations, start by putting the new food on the plate three times, and then touching or licking the new food three times before moving up to three bites.

Resources

2015 Healthy Lunchtime Challenge Cookbook: *https://whatscooking.fns.usda.gov/2015-healthy-lunchtime-challenge-cookbook*

Worksheets, activities, recipes, and healthy eating tips: *www.choosemyplate.gov*

Apps with healthy-eating-related games: Awesome Eats, Healthy Food Monsters

Conclusion

Targeting health behaviors and adherence to medical regimens has many benefits for children and families. In addition to improving the physical health of the child, providing behavioral health interventions around these areas can reduce family conflict and decrease medical costs. Providers working in various settings can utilize the *Express* interventions presented throughout this chapter with the children and families with whom they work. These interventions will help arm providers with strategies to quickly address families' understanding of medical regimens, identify and remove barriers to adherence, and increase overall adherence to the plans, therefore leading to better health outcomes for the children.

Learning about Swallowing

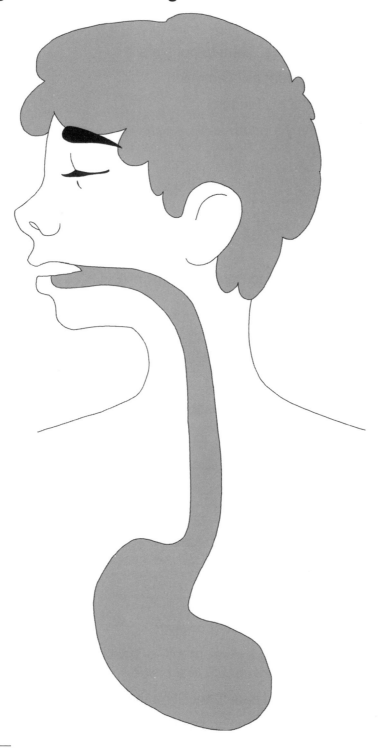

Take It Home: Tips for Swallowing

1. Pill position

For the easiest swallowing, I want to put the pill:

☐ as far back in my throat as I can reach

☐ in the very center of my tongue

☐ on the very tip of my tongue

☐ in the dog's dish

Mark an X on the mouth where the pill should be placed:

2. Drink it down

How big should my sip be to wash down my pill?

☐ just a teeny tiny bit

☐ a regular drink of water

☐ as much as I can fit in my mouth

☐ it's best to swallow the pills dry

Drinks I would like to use when swallowing pills:

a. _____

b. _____

c. _____

Instead of liquid I can try using _____ foods! I want to test out:

a. _____

b. _____

c. _____

3. Head position (circle the correct answer)

If I keep getting the pill stuck in my mouth or my cheeks, I need to try tilting my head *forward* OR *backward* OR *to the side*.

If it feels like I'm choking, I should try tilting my head *forward* OR *backward*.

No matter what direction I'm tilting I always want to do it *a little* OR *a lot*.

Score Card: Sample

Level	My Choices	Score
Itty Bitty	ainbow sprinkles	⊗
Tiny	silver sprinkels	⊗
Small	orange Tic tak	⊗
Medium	Reese's Pieces	\
Large	peanut m&ms	
Extra Credit	NO!	

Homework: 3 Reese's pieces and 3 m+m's

Reward: sleepover with clara!

Score Card

Level	My Choices	Score
Itty Bitty		
Tiny		
Small		
Medium		
Large		
Extra Credit		

Homework:

Reward:

Overcoming Obstacles

You're so close, don't give up! Do some experiments with some of these ideas or make up your own! These ideas will help you overcome the final obstacles to your success.

Try changing . . .

    The beverage being used:

    Stronger flavors are better flavor blockers for pills.

        Our ideas:

            Cherry Kool-aid

            Tart lemonade

            Dr. Pepper

        Your ideas:

_____

_____

    Instead of liquid, use a mushy food like:

    Experiment to see if neutral flavors or preferred flavors work best.

        Our ideas:

            Yogurt

            Mashed potatoes

            Frozen yogurt/ice cream

            Apple sauce

            Cottage cheese

        Your ideas:

_____

_____

    Trick your senses by trying one of these:

    Find something cold or with a really strong flavor that will confuse your mouth.

        Our ideas:

            Suck on a popsicle or ice cube for 5–10 seconds before and after swallowing the pill.

            Suck on a strong mint for 5–10 seconds before and after swallowing the pill.

            Chew cinnamon gum for 5–10 seconds before (remove from mouth), swallow pill, return gum to mouth.

            Suck on a sour candy for 5–10 seconds before and after swallowing the pill.

        Your ideas:

_____

_____

Fast Facts for My Medications: Sample

What my medications are called: (Draw the size and shape next to each one.)	Who gives them to me?
clonidine ⬭ Adderall	I do mom double checks

When do I take them?	Where are my medications kept?
Adderall - at breakfast clonidine- after brush teeth	In the kitchen

Special Instructions: (e.g., with food, 30 minutes before bed)	Why am I taking these? (specific targets)
Adderall has to be in the morning clonidine has to be right before bed	to help me focus and calm down also to help me sleep

How will this help me? (how my life will be different)

I can do my homework faster
My teachers might like me more
I won't get bored when I can't fall asleep

Fast Facts for My Medications

What my medications are called: (Draw the size and shape next to each one.)	Who gives them to me?

When do I take them?	Where are my medications kept?

Special Instructions: (e.g., with food, 30 minutes before bed)	Why am I taking these? (specific targets)

How will this help me? (how my life will be different)

Piece It Together

I Keep My Medicine:

☐ In the kitchen

☐ In _____ bathroom

☐ In _____ bedroom

☐ In my backpack/school bag

☐ In my (or Mom's) purse

The Adult Who Supervises Me Is:

☐ Mom

☐ Dad

☐ Grandparent

☐ Babysitter

☐ _____

We Keep Records On:

☐ A worksheet or calendar posted _____

☐ An app called _____ on _____

We Get Reminders From:

☐ An alarm on _____

☐ A sign on _____

☐ A notification from _____

My Medicine Monitor

Today is: _____

Put a sticker on each day you take medicine.

I come back on: _____   I can earn: _____

Monday	Tuesday	Wednesday	Thursday	Friday	Saturday	Sunday

Helping or Harming?: Sample

In the space below, draw the shape of the medication(s). Color in a portion of the pill to represent how helpful you think this medication is. Using a different color, shade in a portion to represent how harmful this medication is.

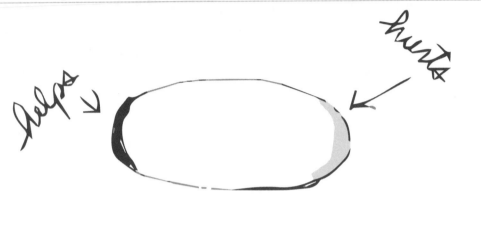

Best possible outcome from taking this medication is:

∅

Worst possible outcome from taking this medication is:

diarrhea
accidents

Helping or Harming?

In the space below, draw the shape of the medication(s). Color in a portion of the pill to represent how helpful you think this medication is. Using a different color, shade in a portion to represent how harmful this medication is.

Best possible outcome from taking this medication is:

Worst possible outcome from taking this medication is:

Test It Out

It's Working!!	No It's Not!
It Works Best When:	**Things That Get in the Way:**

Decision:

Willing to Try?   YES   NO

Green, Yellow, Red

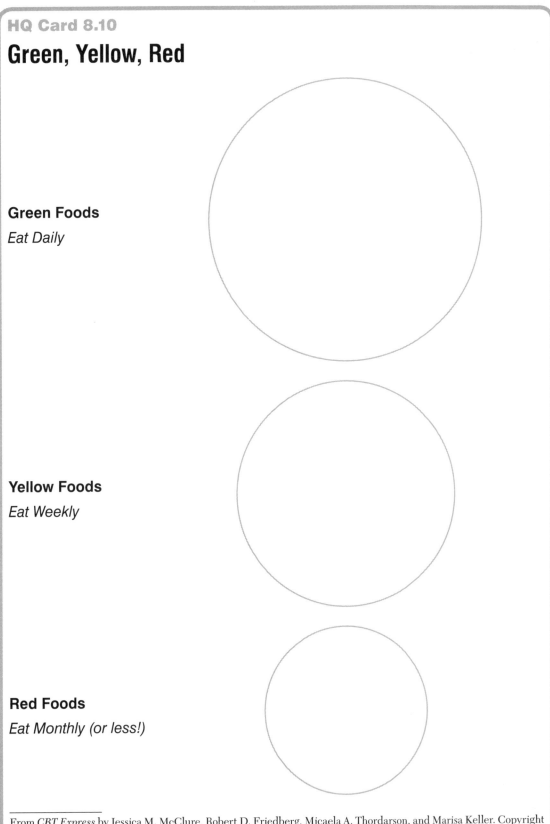

Green Foods

Eat Daily

Yellow Foods

Eat Weekly

Red Foods

Eat Monthly (or less!)

My Shopping List

🙂	🙁
	This Week's Special Treat:

Scavenger Hunt

Draw foods in the places you will find them in your home!

Family Menu

The

_____

Family Menu

BREAKFAST	LUNCH

SNACKS	DINNER

Money-Saving Tips for Healthy Eating

1. Buy whole/unprocessed foods—if it's ready to go, you're paying extra.
   - For example, shredded cheese or prechopped veggies cost more.
   - Oatmeal packets with flavors mixed in cost more than the tub of plain oats.

2. Buy cheap proteins—eggs, plain yogurt, cottage cheese, frozen chicken breast.

3. Eat less meat (but make sure to get protein elsewhere).

4. Buy frozen fruits and vegetables.

5. Buy generic and store brands.

6. Buy in bulk—fruit and meats can be frozen.

7. Buy fruits and vegetables that are in season.

8. Buy everything at one store to save time and gas money.

9. Shop at farmer's markets to buy fresh in-season fruit (showing up later may give you fewer options, but prices are lower too).

10. Clip coupons, but only keep the ones for things you know you will be buying.

11. Sign up for customer rewards programs.

12. Check the unit price at the bottom of the price tag to compare between options for the best deal.

13. Avoid impulse buying.
    - ☐ Make a list before you get to the store so you know exactly what you need.
    - ☐ Plan the meals for the week so you don't end up wasting food (and money).
    - ☐ Shop alone as often as possible, or limit each shopper to a single choice of his or her own.
    - ☐ Don't shop hungry (everything looks like a good idea!).

14. Always pack snacks to cut down on buying food when out and about.

15. Grow your own food! Plant a tree, build a garden box for the patio, or put together a small pot for the kitchen window—however you do it, any little bit helps! Home-grown tastes the best too! ☺

Pros and Cons: Sample (Jaimie's Example)

Let's Do This!   Never Happening

List two to three pros to following the plan.	List two to three cons to following the plan.
+	**—**
• Everyone will quit bothering me about what I eat.	• I don't get to eat ~~any~~ *a lot* of the things I like any more.
• I might feel better.	• I can't eat birthday cake at my friend Taylor's party this weekend.
• I probably won't have to go to the hospital as much.	• My friends ~~will~~ *might* think I'm weird.

Pros and Cons: Sample (Jaimie's Mom's Example)

Let's Do This!   Never Happening

List two to three pros to following the plan.	List two to three cons to following the plan.
+	**—**
• I might feel healthier too. • We will do this together. • It will *probably* be easier for Jaimie if I'm making changes too.	• I have to give up my Diet Coke. • Grocery shopping is going to be harder *for a little while.* • If I sneak chocolate, I will *probably* feel guilty for doing that.

Pros and Cons

Let's Do This!   Never Happening

List two to three pros to following the plan.	List two to three cons to following the plan.
+	**—**

References

Akerof, G. A. (1970). The market for "lemons": Quality uncertainty and the market mechanism. *Quarterly Journal of Economics, 84,* 488–500.

Aldao, A., Nolen-Hoeksema, S., & Schweizer, S. (2010). Emotion-regulation strategies across psychopathology: A meta-analytic review. *Clinical Psychology Review, 30,* 217–237.

Allen, L. B., Ehrenreich, J. T., & Barlow, D. H. (2005). A unified treatment for emotional disorders: Applications with adults and adolescents [invited article]. *Japanese Journal of Behavior Therapy, 31*(1), 3–30.

Arnberg, A., & Ost, L. G. (2014). CBT for children with depressive symptoms: A meta-analysis. *Cognitive Behaviour Therapy, 43*(4), 275–288.

Asarnow, J. R., Hoagwood, K. E., Stancin, T., Lochman, J., Hughes, J. L., Miranda, J. M., et al. (2015). Psychological science and innovative strategies for informing health care redesign: A policy brief. *Journal of Clinical Child and Adolescent Psychology, 44,* 923–932.

Asarnow, J. R., Kolko, D. J., Miranda, J., & Kazak, A. (2017). The pediatric patient-centered medical home: Innovative models for improving behavioral health. *American Psychologist, 72,* 13–27.

Barker, S. L. (1983). Supply side economics in private psychotherapy practice: Some ominous and encouraging trends. *Psychotherapy in Private Practice, 1,* 71–81.

Beauchaine, T. P., Hinshaw, S. P., & Pang, K. L. (2010). Comorbidity of attention deficit/hyperactivity disorder and early-onset conduct disorder: Biological, environmental, and developmental mechanisms. *Clinical Psychology: Science and Practice, 17,* 327–336.

Beck, A. T. (1976). *Cognitive therapy and the emotional disorders.* New York: International Universities Press.

Beck, J. S. (2011). *Cognitive behavior therapy: Basics and beyond* (2nd ed.). New York: Guilford Press.

Beidas, R. S., Stewart, R. E., Walsh, L., Lucas, S., Downey, M. M., Jackson, K., et al. (2015). Free, brief, and validated: Standardized instruments for low-resource mental health settings. *Cognitive and Behavioral Practice, 22,* 5–19.

Bennett, K., Manassis, K., Duda, S., Bagnell, A., Bernstein, G. A., Garland, E. J., et al. (2016). Treating child and adolescent anxiety effectively: Overview of systematic reviews. *Clinical Psychology Review, 50,* 80–94.

Berry, R. R., & Lai, B. (2014). The emerging role of technology in cognitive–behavioral therapy for anxious youth: A review. *Journal of Rational-Emotive and Cognitive-Behavior Therapy, 32*(1), 57–66.

Bickman, L. (2008). A measurement feedback system (MFS) is necessary to improve mental health outcomes. *Journal of the American Academy of Child and Adolescent Psychiatry, 47,* 1114–1119.

Bickman, L., Douglas-Kelley, S., Breda, C., de Andrade, A. R., & Reimer, M. (2011). Effects of routine feedback to clinicians on mental health outcomes of youths: Results of a randomized trial. *Psychiatric Services, 62,* 1423–1429.

Brinkmeyer, M. Y., & Eyberg, S. M. (2003). Parent–child interaction therapy for oppositional children. In A. E. Kazdin & J. R. Weisz (Eds.), *Evidence-based psychotherapies for children and adolescents* (pp. 204–223). New York: Guilford Press.

Campo, J. V., Shafer, S., Strohm, J., Lucas, A., Gelacek-Cassesse, C., Saheffer, D., et al. (2005). Pediatric behavioral health in primary care: A collaborative approach. *Journal of the American Psychiatric Nurses Association, 11,* 276–282.

Carlson, C. R., & Hoyle, R. H. (1993). Efficacy of abbreviated progressive muscle relaxation training: A quantitative review of behavioral medicine research. *Journal of Consulting and Clinical Psychology, 61,* 1059–1067.

Carthy, T., Horesch, N., Apter, A., Edge, M. D., & Gross, J. J. (2010). Emotional reactivity and cognitive regulation in anxious children. *Behaviour Research and Therapy, 48,* 384–393.

Chess, S., & Thomas, A. (1999). *Goodness of fit: Clinical applications from infancy through adult life.* Philadelphia: Brunner/Mazel.

Cho, Y., & Telch, M. J. (2005). Testing the cognitive content-specificity hypothesis of social anxiety and depression: An application of structural equation modeling. *Cognitive Therapy and Research, 29,* 399–416.

Chorpita, B., & Daleiden, E. (2009). Mapping evidence-based treatments for children and adolescents: Applications of the distillation and matching model to 615 treatments from 322 randomized trials. *Journal of Consulting and Clinical Psychology, 77,* 566–579.

Chorpita, B. F., Daleiden, E. L., & Weisz, J. R. (2005). Identifying and selecting the common elements of evidence based interventions: A distillation and matching model. *Mental Health Services Research, 7*(1), 5–20.

Chorpita, B. F., & Weisz, J. R. (2009). *MATCH-ADTC: Modular approach to therapy for children with anxiety, depression, trauma, or conduct problems.* Satellite Beach, FL: Practice-Wise.

Christopherson, E. R., & Mortweet, S. L. (2013). *Treatments that work with children: Empirically suggested strategies for managing problem* (2nd ed.). Washington, DC: American Psychological Association.

Clarke, G., Debar, L., Lynch, F., Powell, J., Gale, J., O'Connor, E., et al. (2005). A randomized effectiveness trial of brief cognitive-behavioral therapy for depressed adolescents receiving antidepressant medication. *Journal of the American Academy of Child and Adolescent Psychiatry, 44*(9), 888–898.

Cone, J. D. (1997). Issues in functional analysis in behavioral assessment. *Behaviour Research and Therapy, 35,* 259–275.

Cooper, J. O., Heron, T. E., & Heward, W. L. (Eds.). (1987). *Applied behavioral analysis.* New York: Macmillan.

Cortina, S., Somers, M., Rohan, J. M., & Drotar, D. (2013). Clinical effectiveness of comprehensive psychological intervention for nonadherence to medical treatment: A case series. *Journal of Pediatric Psychology, 38*(6), 649–663.

Cox, G. R., Fisher, C. A., DeSilva, S., Phelan, M., Akinwale, O. P., Simmons, M. B., et al. (2012). Interventions for preventing relapse and recurrence of depressive disorder in children and adolescents. *Cochrane Database of Systematic Reviews, 11,* CD007504.

Crawley, S. A., Kendall, P. C., Benjamin, C. L., Brodman, D. M., Wei, C., Beidas, R. S., et al. (2013). Brief cognitive-behavioral therapy for anxious youth: Feasibility and initial outcomes. *Cognitive and Behavioral Practice, 20*(2), 123–133.

Curry, J. F., & Wells, K. C. (2005). Striving for effectiveness in the treatment of adolescent depression: Cognitive behavior therapy for multisite community intervention. *Cognitive and Behavioral Practice, 12,* 177–185.

David-Ferdon, C., & Kaslow, N. J. (2008). Evidence-based psychosocial treatments for child and adolescent depression. *Journal of Clinical Child and Adolescent Psychology, 37*(1), 62–104.

Dodge, K. A. (2006). Translational science in action: Hostile attributional style and the development of aggressive behavior problems. *Development and Psychopathology, 18,* 791–814.

Drayton, A. K., Andersen, M. N., Knight, R. M., Felt, B. T., Fredericks, E. M., & Dore-Stiles, D. J. (2012). Internet guidance on time-out: Inaccuracies, omissions, and what to tell parents instead. *Journal of Developmental and Behavioral Pediatrics, 35,* 239–246.

Ehrenreich, J. T., Goldstein, C. R., Wright, L. R., & Barlow, D. H. (2009). Development of a unified protocol for the treatment of emotional disorders in youth. *Child and Family Behavior Therapy, 31,* 20–37.

Elkins, R. M., McHugh, R. K., Santucci, L. C., & Barlow, D. H. (2011). Improving the transportability of CBT for internalizing disorders in children. *Clinical Child and Family Psychology Review, 14*(2), 161–173.

Eyberg, S. M., Nelson, M. M., & Boggs, S. R. (2008). Evidence-based psychosocial treatments for children and adolescents with disruptive behavior. *Journal of Clinical Child and Adolescent Psychology, 37,* 215–237.

Flessner, C. A., & Piacentini, J. C. (Eds.). (2017). *Clinical handbook of psychological disorders in children and adolescents.* New York: Guilford Press.

Forehand, R., & McMahon, R. J. (1981). *Helping the noncompliant child: A clinician's guide to parent training.* New York: Guilford Press.

Frick, P. J., & Morris, A. S. (2004). Temperament and developmental pathways to conduct problems. *Journal of Clinical Child and Adolescent Psychology, 33,* 54–68.

Friedberg, R. D. (2015). When treatment as usual gives you lemons, count on evidence based practices. *Child and Family Behavior Therapy, 37,* 335–348.

Friedberg, R. D., & Brelsford, G. M. (2011). Using cognitive behavioral interventions to help children cope with parental military deployments. *Journal of Contemporary Psychotherapy, 41,* 229–236.

Friedberg, R. D., Gorman, A. A., Hollar-Wilt, L. H., Biuckians, A., & Murray, M. (2012). *Cognitive behavioral therapy for the busy child psychiatrist and other mental health professionals: Rubrics and rudiments.* New York: Routledge.

Friedberg, R. D., & McClure, J. M. (2015). *Clinical practice of cognitive therapy with children and adolescents: The nuts and bolts* (2nd ed.). New York: Guilford Press.

Friedberg, R. D., McClure, J. M., & Hillwig-Garcia, J. (2009). *Cognitive therapy techniques for children and adolescents: Tools for enhancing practice.* New York: Guilford Press.

Friedberg, R. D., & Rozbruch, E. V. (2016). Quality counts: Behavioral health care services with youth should be guided by outcome metrics. *Clinical Psychiatry, 2,* 1–2.

Friedberg, R. D., Thordarson, M. A., Paternostro, J., Sullivan, P., & Tamas, M. (2014). CBT with youth: Immodest proposals for training the next generation. *Journal of Rational-Emotive and Cognitive Behavior Therapy, 32,* 110–119.

Ghahramanlou-Holloway, M., Wenzel, A., Lou, K., & Beck, A. T. (2007). Differentiating cognitive content between depressed and anxious outpatients. *Cognitive Behavioral Therapy, 36,* 170–178.

Goldstein, N. E., Serico, J. M., Romaine, C. L. R., Zelechoski, A. D., Kalbeitzer, R., Kemp, K., et al. (2013). Development of the juvenile justice anger management treatment for girls. *Cognitive and Behavioral Practice, 20*(2), 171–188.

Görzig, A., & Frumkin, L. A. (2013). Cyberbullying experiences on-the-go: When social media can become distressing. *Cyberpsychology: Journal of Psychosocial Research on Cyberspace, 7*(1).

Gross, J. J. (1998). The emerging field of emotion regulation: An integrative review. *Review of General Psychology, 2*(3), 271–299.

Hammond, W. R., & Yung, B. R. (1991). Preventing violence in at-risk African-American youth. *Journal of Health Care for the Poor and Underserved, 2*(3), 359–373.

Hankinson, J. C., & Slifer, K. J. (2013). Behavioral treatments to improve pill swallowing and adherence in an adolescent with renal and connective tissue diseases. *Clinical Practice in Pediatric Psychology, 1*(3), 227–234.

Hannesdottir, D. K., & Ollendick, T. H. (2007). The role of emotion regulation in the treatment of child anxiety disorders. *Clinical Child and Family Psychology Review, 10,* 275–293.

Haynes, S. N., O'Brien, W., & Kaholokula, J. (2011). *Behavioral assessment and case formulation.* New York: Wiley.

Henggeler, S. W., & Lee, T. (2003). Multisystemic treatment of serious clinical problems. In A. E. Kazdin & J. R. Weisz (Eds.), *Evidence-based psychotherapies for children and adolescents* (pp. 301–322). New York: Guilford Press.

Higa-McMillan, C. K., Francis, S. E., Rith-Najarian, L., & Chorpita, B. F. (2016). Evidence base update: 50 years of research on treatment for child and adolescent anxiety. *Journal of Clinical Child and Adolescent Psychology, 45*(2), 91–113.

Janicke, D. M., Fritz, A. M., & Rozensky, R. M. (2015). Healthcare reform and preparing the future clinical child and adolescent psychology workforce. *Journal of Clinical Child and Adolescent Psychology, 44,* 1030–1039.

Kazdin, A. E. (2001). *Behavior modification in applied settings.* Belmont, CA: Wadsworth.

Kazdin, A. E. (2008). *The Kazdin method for parenting the defiant child.* Boston: Houghton Mifflin.

Kazdin, A. E. (2010). Problem-solving skills training and parent management training for oppositional defiant disorder and conduct disorder. In J. R. Weisz & A. E. Kazdin (Eds.), *Evidence-based psychotherapies for children and adolescents* (2nd ed., pp. 211–226). New York: Guilford Press.

Kendall, P. C. (Ed.). (2017). *Cognitive therapy with children and adolescents: A casebook for clinical practice* (3rd ed.). New York: Guilford Press.

Kendall, P. C., & Peterman, J. S. (2015). CBT for adolescents with anxiety: Mature yet still developing. *American Journal of Psychiatry, 172*(6), 519–530.

Kennard, B. D., Emslie, G. J., Mayes, T. L., Nightingale-Teresi, J., Nakonezny, P. A., Hughes, J. L., et al. (2008). Cognitive-behavioral therapy to prevent relapse in pediatric responders to pharmacotherapy for major depressive disorder. *Journal of the American Academy of Child and Adolescent Psychiatry, 47*(12), 1395–1404.

Kennard, B. D., Hughes, J. L., & Foxwell, A. A. (2016). *CBT for depression in children and adolescents: A guide to relapse prevention.* New York: Guilford Press.

Kirch, D. G., & Ast, C. E. (2017). Health care transformation: The role of academic health centers and their psychologists. *Journal of Clinical Psychology in Medical Settings, 24*(2), 86–91.

Kuyken, W., Padesk, C. A., & Dudley, R. (2008). *Collaborative case conceptualization.* New York: Guilford Press.

Lambert, M. J., Whipple, J. L., Vermeersch, D. A., Smart, D. W., Hawkins, E. J., Nielsen, S. L., et al. (2002). Enhancing psychotherapy outcomes via providing feedback on client progress: A replication. *Clinical Psychology and Psychotherapy, 9,* 91–103.

Lamberton, A., & Oei, T. P. (2008). A test of the cognitive content specificity hypothesis in depression and anxiety. *Journal of Behavior Therapy and Experimental Psychiatry, 39,* 23–31.

Landenberger, N. A., & Lipsey, M. W. (2005). The positive effects of cognitive–behavioral programs for offenders: A meta-analysis of factors associated with effective treatment. *Journal of Experimental Criminology, 1*(4), 451–476.

Lavigne, J. V., Gouze, K. R., Hopkins, J., Bryant, F. B., & LeBailly, S. A. (2012). A multi-domain model of risk factors for ODD symptoms in a community sample of 4-year-olds. *Journal of Abnormal Child Psychology, 40,* 741–757.

Linehan, M. M. (1993). *Cognitive-behavioral treatment of borderline personality disorder.* New York: Guilford Press.

Linehan, M. M. (2014). *DBT® skills training manual.* New York: Guilford Press.

Lochman, J. E., Powell, N. P., Boxmeyer, C. L., & Jimenez-Camargo, L. (2011). Cognitive-behavioral therapy for externalizing disorders in children and adolescents. *Child and Adolescent Psychiatry Clinics of North America, 20,* 305–318.

Lochman, J. E., & Wells, K. C. (2002). Contextual social-cognitive mediators and child outcome: A test of the theoretical model in the Coping Power program. *Development and Psychopathology, 14*(4), 945–967.

Lochman, J. E., & Wells, K. C. (2003). Effectiveness of the Coping Power program and of classroom intervention with aggressive children: Outcomes at a 1-year follow-up. *Behavior Therapy, 34*(4), 493–515.

Lochman, J. E., & Wells, K. C. (2004). The Coping Program for preadolescent aggressive boys and their parents: Outcome effects at the 1-year follow-up. *Journal of Consulting and Clinical Psychology, 72,* 571–578.

Luersen, K., Davis, S. A., Kaplan, S. G., Abel, T. D., Winchester, W. W., & Feldman, S. R. (2012). Sticker charts: A method for improving adherence to treatment of chronic diseases in children. *Pediatric Dermatology, 29*(4), 403–408.

Manassis, K. (2009). *CBT with children: A guide for the community practitioner.* New York: Routledge.

Manassis, K. (2012). *Problem solving in child and adolescent psychotherapy: A skills-based, collaborative approach.* New York: Guilford Press.

Manassis, K. (2014). *Case formulation with children and adolescents.* New York: Guilford Press.

March, J., Silva, S., Petrycki, S., Curry, J., Wells, K., Fairbank, J., et al. (2004). Fluoxetine, cognitive-behavioral therapy, and their combination for adolescents with depression: Treatment for Adolescents with Depression Study (TADS) randomized controlled trial. *JAMA, 292*(7), 807–820.

Martel, M. M., Gremillion, M. L., & Roberts, B. (2012). Temperament and common disruptive behavior problems in preschool. *Personality and Individual Differences, 53,* 874–879.

Martinez, C. R., Jr., & Eddy, J. M. (2005). Effects of culturally adapted parent management training on Latino youth behavioral health outcomes. *Journal of Consulting and Clinical Psychology, 73*(5), 841–851.

McCart, M. R., & Sheidow, A. J. (2016). Evidence-based psychosocial treatments for adolescents with disruptive behavior. *Journal of Clinical Child and Adolescent Psychology, 45*(5), 529–563.

McCauley, E., Schloredt, K., Gudmundsen, G., Martell, C., & Dimidjian, S. (2011). Expanding behavioral activation to depressed adolescents: Lessons learned in treatment development. *Cognitive and Behavioral Practice, 18*(3), 371–383.

McGrady, M. E., Ryan, J. L., Brown, G. A., & Cushing, C. C. (2015). Topical review: Theoretical frameworks in pediatric adherence-promotion interventions: Research findings and methodological implications. *Journal of Pediatric Psychology, 40*(8), 721–726.

McLaughlin, K. A., Hatzenbuehler, M. L., Mennin, D. S., & Nolen-Hoeksema, S. (2011). Emotion dysregulation and adolescent psychopathology: A prospective study. *Behavioral Research and Therapy, 49*(9), 544–554.

McLeod, B. D., Jensen-Doss, A., & Ollendick, T. H. (Eds.). (2013). *Diagnostic and behavioral assessment in children and adolescents: A clinical guide.* New York: Guilford Press.

Meltzer, E. O., Welch, M. J., & Ostrom, N. K. (2006). Pill swallowing ability and training in children 6 to 11 years of age. *Clinical Pediatrics, 45*(8), 725–733.

Melvin, G. A., Tonge, B. J., King, N. J., Heyne, D., Gordon, M. S., & Klimkeit, E. (2006). A comparison of cognitive-behavioral therapy, sertraline, and their combination for adolescent depression. *Journal of the American Academy of Child and Adolescent Psychiatry, 45*(10), 1151–1161.

Miller, A. (2015, November). *The business of CBT.* Workshop presented at the annual meeting of the Association for Behavioral and Cognitive Therapies, Chicago, IL.

Miller, A. L., Rathus, J. H., & Linehan, M. M. (2006). *Dialectical behavior therapy with suicidal adolescents.* New York: Guilford Press.

Modi, A. C., Guilfoyle, S. M., & Rausch, J. (2013). Preliminary feasibility, acceptability, and efficacy of an innovative adherence intervention for children with newly diagnosed epilepsy. *Journal of Pediatric Psychology, 38*(6), 605–616.

Muris, P., & Ollendick, T. H. (2005). The role of temperament in the etiology of child psychopathology. *Clinical Child and Family Psychology Review, 8*(4), 271–289.

Nangle, D. W., Hansen, D. J., Grover, R. L., Kingery, J. N., Suveg, C., & Contributors. (2016). *Treating internalizing disorders in children and adolescents: Core techniques and strategies.* New York: Guilford Press.

Nock, M. K., Kazdin, A. E., Hiripi, E., & Kessler, R. C. (2007). Lifetime prevalence, correlates, and persistence of oppositional defiant disorder: Results from the National Comorbidity Survey Replication. *Journal of Child Psychology and Psychiatry, 48*, 703–713.

Osmanoglou, E., Voort, I. R., Fach, K., Kosch, O., Bach, D., Hartmann, V., et al. (2004). Oesophageal transport of solid dosage forms depends on body position, swallowing volume and pharyngeal propulsion velocity. *Neurogastroenterology and Motility, 16*(5), 547–556.

Patterson, G. R, Reid, J. B., Jones, R. R., & Conger, R. E. (1975). *A social learning approach: Families with aggressive children* (Vol. 1). Eugene, OR: Castalia.

Pereira, A. I., Muris, P., Mendonça, D., Barros, L., Goes, A. R., & Marques, T. (2016). Parental involvement in cognitive-behavioral intervention for anxious children: Parents' in-session and out-session activities and their relationship with treatment outcome. *Child Psychiatry and Human Development, 47*(1), 113–123.

Persons, J. B. (2008). *The case formulation approach to cognitive-behavioral therapy.* New York: Guilford Press.

Peterman, J. S., Carper, M. M., Elkins, R. M., Comer, J. S., Pincus, D. B., & Kendall, P. C. (2016). The effects of cognitive-behavioral therapy for youth anxiety on sleep problems. *Journal of Anxiety Disorders, 37*, 78–88.

Rapoff, M. A. (2010). *Adherence to pediatric medical regimens.* New York: Springer Science+Business Media.

Reyes-Portillo, J. A., Mufson, L., Greenhill, L. L., Gould, M. S., Fisher, P. W., Tarlow, N., et al. (2014). Web-based interventions for youth internalizing problems: A systematic review. *Journal of the American Academy of Child and Adolescent Psychiatry, 53*(12), 1254–1270.

Roberts, M. C., Aylward, B. S., & Wu, Y. P. (Eds.). (2014). *Clinical practice of pediatric psychology.* New York: Guilford Press.

Robinson, T. R., Smith, S. W., & Miller, M. D. (1999). Cognitive behavior modification of hyperactivity-impulsivity and aggression: A meta-analysis of school-based studies. *Journal of Educational Psychology, 91*, 195–203.

Rosselló, J., Bernal, G., & Rivera-Medina, C. (2012). Individual and group CBT and IPT for Puerto Rican adolescents with depressive symptoms. *Cultural Diversity and Ethnic Minority Psychology, 14*(3), 234–245.

Rudolph, K. D., & Troop-Gordon, W. (2010). Personal-accentuation and contextual-amplification models of pubertal timing: Predicting youth depression. *Development and Psychopathology, 22*(2), 433–451.

Sandil, R. (2006). Cognitive behavioral therapy for adolescent depression: Implications for Asian immigrants in the United States of America. *Journal of Child and Adolescent Mental Health, 18*(1), 27–32.

Sburlati, E. S., Lyneham, H. J., Schniering, C. A., & Rapee, R. M. (Eds.). (2016). *Evidence-based CBT for anxiety and depression in adolescence.* West Sussex, UK: Wiley.

Schiele, J. T., Schneider, H., Quinzler, R., Reich, G., & Haefeli, W. E. (2014). Two techniques to make swallowing pills easier. *Annals of Family Medicine, 12*(6), 550–552.

Schniering, C. A., & Rapee, R. M. (2002). Development and validation of a measure of children's automatic thoughts: The Children's Automatic Thoughts Scale. *Behaviour Research and Therapy, 40*, 1091–1109.

Scott, K., & Lewis, C. C. (2015). Using measurement-based care to enhance any treatment. *Cognitive and Behavioral Practice, 22*(1), 49–59.

Seligman, L. D., & Ollendick, T. H. (2011). Cognitive-behavioral therapy for anxiety disorders in youth. *Child and Adolescent Psychiatric Clinics of North America, 20*(2), 217–238.

Serrano, N., Cordes, C., Cubic, B., & Daub, S. (2018). The state and future of the primary care behavioral health model of service delivery workforce.

Journal of Clinical Psychology in Medical Settings, 25(2), 157–168.

Simons, A. D., Marti, C. N., Rohde, P., Lewis, C. C., Curry, J., & March, J. (2012). Does homework "matter" in cognitive behavioral therapy for adolescent depression? *Journal of Cognitive Psychotherapy, 26*(4), 390–404.

Smith, S. W., Lochman, J. E., & Daunic, A. P. (2005). Managing aggression using cognitive-behavioral interventions: State of the practice and future directions. *Behavioral Disorders, 30*(3), 227–240.

Southam-Gerow, M. A. (2016). *Emotion regulation in children and adolescents: A practitioner's guide.* New York: Guilford Press

Southam-Gerow, M. A., & Kendall, P. C. (2002). Emotion regulation and understanding: Implications for child psychopathology and therapy. *Clinical Psychology Review, 22*, 189–222.

Spirito, A., Esposito-Smythers, C., Wolff, J., & Uhl, K. (2011). Cognitive-behavioral therapy for adolescent depression and suicidality. *Child and Adolescent Psychiatric Clinics of North America, 20*(2), 191–204.

Stice, E., Rohde, P., Seeley, J. R., & Gau, J. M. (2008). Brief cognitive-behavioral depression prevention program for high-risk adolescents outperforms two alternative interventions: A randomized efficacy trial. *Journal of Consulting and Clinical Psychology, 76*(4), 595–606.

Sukhodolsky, D. G., Kassinove, H., & Gorman, B. S. (2004). Cognitive-behavioral therapy for anger in children and adolescents: A meta-analysis. *Aggressive and Violent Behavior, 9*, 247–269.

Suveg, C., Morelen, D., Brewer, G. A., & Thomassin, K. (2010). The emotion dysregulation model of anxiety: A preliminary path analytic examination. *Journal of Anxiety Disorders, 24*, 924–930.

Tiwari, S., Kendall, P. C., Hoff, A. L., Harrison, J. P., & Fizur, P. (2013). Characteristics of exposure sessions as predictors of treatment response in anxious youth. *Journal of Clinical Child and Adolescent Psychology, 42*(1), 34–43.

Unutzer, J., Chan, Y.-F., Hafer, E., Knaster, Shields, A., Powers, D., et al. (2012). Quality improvement with pay-for-performance incentives in integrated behavioral health care. *American Journal of Public Health, 102*, e41–e45.

Waldman, I. D., Tackett, J. L., Van Hulle, C. A., Applegate, B., Pardini, D., Frick, P. J., et al. (2011). Child and adolescent conduct disorder substantially shares genetic influences with three socioemotional dispositions. *Journal of Abnormal Psychology, 120*, 57–70.

Walkup, J. T., Albano, A. M., Piacentini, J., Birmaher, B., Compton, S. N., Sherrill, J. T., et al. (2008). Cognitive behavioral therapy, sertraline, or a combination in childhood anxiety. *New England Journal of Medicine, 359*(26), 2753–2766.

Webster-Stratton, C., & Reid, M. (2003). The incredible years parents, teachers, and children training series: A multifaceted treatment approach for young children with conduct problems. In A. E. Kazdin & J. R. Weisz (Eds.), *Evidenced-based psychotherapies for children and adolescents* (pp. 224–240). New York: Guilford Press.

Weersing, V. R., Jeffreys, M., Do, M. C. T., Schwartz, K. T., & Bolano, C. (2017). Evidence base update of psychosocial treatments for child and adolescent depression. *Journal of Clinical Child and Adolescent Psychology, 46*(1), 11–43.

Weersing, V. R., Rozenman, M. S., Maher-Bridge, M., & Campo, J. V. (2012). Anxiety, depression, and somatic distress: Developing a transdiagnostic internalizing toolbox for pediatric practice. *Cognitive and Behavioral Practice, 19*(1), 68–82.

Weersink, R. A., Taxis, K., McGuire, T. M., & van Driel, M. L. (2015). Consumers' questions about antipsychotic medication: Revealing safety concerns and the silent voices of young men. *Social Psychiatry and Psychiatric Epidemiology, 50*(5), 725–733.

Weisz, J. R., & Kazdin, A. E. (Eds.). (2017). *Evidence-based psychotherapies for children and adolescents* (3rd ed.). New York: Guilford Press.

Weitzman, C. C., & Leventhal, J. M. (2006). Screening for behavioral health problems in primary care. *Current Opinions in Pediatrics, 18*, 641–648.

Wolff, J. C., & Ollendick, T. H. (2010). Conduct problems in youth: Phenomenology classification, and epidemiology. In R. C. Murrihy, A. D. Kidman, & T. H. Ollendick (Eds.), *Clinical handbook of assessing and treating conduct problems in youth* (pp. 3–20). New York: Springer.

Wu, Y. P., Rohan, J. M., Martin, S., Hommel, K., Greenley, R. N., Loiselle, K., et al. (2013). Pediatric psychologist use of adherence assessments and interventions. *Journal of Pediatric Psychology, 38*(6), 595–604.

Index

Note. *f* following a page number indicates a figure.